DENTISTS
AT WAR

Major V. H. Ward

UPFRONT PUBLISHING
LEICESTERSHIRE

DENTISTS AT WAR
Copyright © Major V. H. Ward 1996
Copyright © The Army Medical Services Museum 2004

ISBN 1-84426-277-4

First published in 1996 and 1998 by
MINERVA PRESS

Second edition published 2004 by
UPFRONT PUBLISHING LTD
Leicestershire

Printed by Lightning Source

DENTISTS AT WAR

This book has been assembled from material made available from the Royal Army Dental Corps Museum archive, by kind permission of the Director, Army Dental Service. In commemoration of the fiftieth anniversary of the end of World War Two, dedication is made to those who served in that war but particularly to those that survived to 'tell the tale' herein.

Dentists At War is about men and women, qualified as dental surgeons who were commissioned, either voluntarily or through conscription, into the Army Dental Corps and subsequently into the Royal Army Dental Corps. Their service and experiences went sometimes beyond their calling. They became heroes in extraordinary circumstances, not only in action but also when incarcerated within prisoner-of-war camps.

Although the Corps was not formed until 1921, an active military dental service did exist from the seventeenth century to much later, when civilian volunteer dentists went to South Africa to treat British troops in the Boer War. There were also qualified surgeons commissioned into other Arms and Corps in the Great War 1914-1918 and up to 1921.

This book, however, is dedicated to the officers of the Army Dental Corps in World War Two.

Dentists At War is funded by the Royal Army Dental Corps Association members, who have agreed to donate all sales profits to the Royal Army Dental Corps Benevolent Fund.

Contents

Illustrations

SEVENTEENTH CENTURY DENTAL TREATMENT IN THE CIVIL WAR

Prologue

On the downfall of the Commonwealth in 1660, the various forces in the three kingdoms, numbering some 80,000 men, were entirely disbanded and a small standing army of 5,000 was formed under Charles II. The temporary company surgeon was replaced by a regimental 'Chirurgeon' permanently attached to the regiment, supplying a chest of which no details are available but in which some dental instruments were included, no doubt.

Richard Wiseman, 'the Father of English Surgery', and most noted military surgeon of the Restoration, gives us two important army cases and also a vivid picture of oral surgery at that time, in his great work *Severall Chirurgicall Treatises, 1676*.

Here is one of the army casualties:

> ...One was shot in the face betwixt the Nose and eye on the right side into the Ethmoides by pistol-bullet. After he had been cared some years of the external wound in his face, he became troubled with a fretting Ichor, which discharged by that Nostril; and especially at his first raising in the morning out of Bed it would ran half a spoonful of yellowish colour, which had made a chop or gutter at the lower end of that Nostril by its acrimony. After some years he felt, upon bending his head backward or forewards, the bullet to rowl to and fro over the roof of his mouth.
>
> He complained to me of his grievance at the Hague in Holland, a little before His Majesty's going into

Scotland. We resolv'd Upon the cutting thro' the Palat-bone, to which I placed him in a clear light, one holding his head steady, while I cut into the roof. But the flesh was so close tied to the bone that it would not yield to my spatula as I expected; wherefore I applied a bit of a Caustick-stone and held it to the place with a pledget of lint for a few minutes; by which I consumed the soft fleshy part over the bone, and afterwards cut into the bone such a hole, that in the moving of his head I could see the bullet lodged in the hole; which encouraging us to proceed in our work, the bullet was afterwards taken out, and he eased of that discharge of matter which threaten'd a filthy carious ulcer. My attendance upon His Majesty into Scotland hindering my prosecution of that cure, I left him in the hands of a Chirurgeon there, and since have often seen him at Court. But the Ulcer did not close up with a callus; however the place is supplied by a small plate without offence...

CARTOON IN THE REGIMENT JOURNAL PORTRAYING A VIEW OF MILITARY DENTISTRY

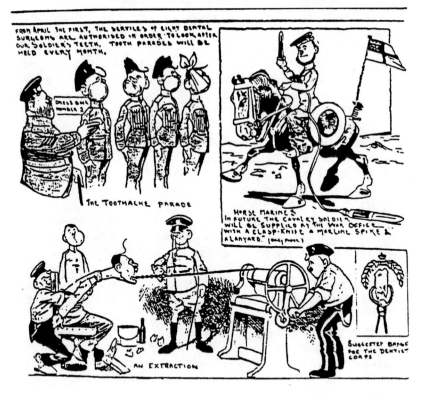

THE BOER WAR, 1899–1902

Prologue

In 1899, two corps of infantry, together with a cavalry division were sent to South Africa to quell the Boer uprising.

During the period of this campaign, the size of the expeditionary force, increasing to 250,000 men, took the field, and operations were conducted under the spotlight of public knowledge. Press correspondents, backed by photography and telegraphed news and letters sent back home from the troops, highlighted the problems of the day. One of these problems was the sick wastage due to dental disease.

While medical arrangements were inadequate, dental arrangements were non-existent. There were no dentists with the original force. Medical Officers of the RAMC did what they could. Some troops were fortunate enough to be stationed in areas where civilian dentists were in practice and were prepared to provide treatment privately.

The diet of the troops was based on beef and biscuits. Oxen were driven to be slaughtered as necessary, but the combination of tough beef and hard biscuits had a disastrous effect on both natural and artificial teeth. At the same time, the drinking of polluted water led to massive outbreaks of enteric and dysentery. The rate of sick to wounded in the campaign was twenty to one. The sick wastage due to dental disease was of such proportions that attention was inevitably drawn to the state of the soldiers' teeth.

An Imperial Yeomanry Hospital was formed and equipped by voluntary subscription. The senior surgeon, Alfred Fripp, decided to include a dentist in the unit and he asked Frederick Newland Pedley, also of Guy's Hospital, to go with him. Pedley sailed from Southampton in February 1900.

The hospital was located at Deelfontein and it was there that he became the first dentist to treat British troops in the field. Working first under canvas then in a hut, he provided his own equipment and

materials and was able to fill teeth, perform extractions under nitrous
oxide, and make a few dentures from materials to hand.

As a result of his situation report, four civilian dental surgeons
were despatched in the following year to treat troops in the field.

Dentures could not be supplied and the majority of extractions had
to be performed without an anaesthetic. The inadequacy of this first
attempt to provide a dental service for a British Army in the field is
shown by the large number that were invalided home as unfit for
service on account of dental caries alone – approximately one-third of
the total admissions to hospital for dental caries (6,942) were
subsequently discharged – a serious loss to the service.

No records exist of the number of men who were evacuated for
'diseases attributable to dental causes', but the total number of dental
sick wastage must have been a considerable strain upon army
resources.

FORMATION WARRANT OF THE ARMY DENTAL CORPS

<u>OFFICIAL COPY</u>

Crown Copyright Reserved

SPECIAL ARMY ORDER
No. 4

THE WAR OFFICE,

11th January, 1921

ROYAL WARRANT

A.O. 4.

1921

Army Dental Corps

GEORGE R.I.

24

;en. No.

7623

WHEREAS WE deem it expedient to authorize the formation of a Corps to be entitled "The Army Dental Corps";

OUR WILL AND PLEASURE IS that Our Army Dental Corps shall be deemed to be a Corps for the purpose of the Army Act and that the words "Army Dental Corps" shall be inserted in Our Warrant of 7th July, 1916,* defining the expression Corps.

OUR FURTHER WILL AND PLEASURE IS that the conditions of service and of promotion and the rates of pay and half-pay and the rates and conditions of retired pay and gratuity of officers, non-commissioned officers and men of Our Army Dental Corps shall be as provided in the schedule attached to this Our Warrant.

Given at Our Court at St. James's, this 4th day of January, 1921, in the 11th year of Our Reign.

By His Majesty's Command,

Winston Churchill (signature)

*Army Order 250 of 1916

THE ARMY DENTAL CORPS

The Army Dental Corps was formed in 1921, this being a very inappropriate time to initiate a new corps to the army.

Politicians, the national press and public opinion had turned their thoughts to rebuilding the ravaged economy of Britain, after the First World War. The Defence budget was never adequate and the public image of dentists or dentistry, even with the passing of the 1921 *Dentists Act*, still was not very high.

It is impossible to indicate in words how far dental treatment helped to prevent wastage of manpower, raise the standard of health, efficiency and morale of the army. The records show that there were over 20,000,000 attendances for treatment, 14,000,000 scalings, 910,000 dentures supplied, 800,000 dentures repaired or remodelled, and at least 15,000 maxillo-facial wounds were treated during the six years of World War Two.

The cost in lives of members of the corps must be mentioned. Thirty-two officers and forty-two other ranks were killed or died on active service. Many were invalided out of the army due to wounds or sickness, and nearly one hundred were held prisoner of war, some under the most appalling conditions.

In November 1914 the first dental officers were commissioned, twelve in number – rising to three hundred by August 1916. May of that year saw these dental officers becoming mechanised – they were presented with a motor dental laboratory, which proved so successful that a further four were issued, one for each of the five armies in France at that time.

By November 1918 there were 850 dental officers serving. These were quickly run down at the end of hostilities, until only a nucleus remained. It was from this nucleus that the Army Dental Corps was formed on the 4th January 1921 with a strength of 110 officers and 132 other ranks. This grew steadily to 237 officers and 326 ORs by the outbreak of the Second World War, expansion keeping pace with the demand throughout the conflict.

TRENCH WARFARE – ROLLS-ROYCE SURGERY

In the Great War of 1914-1918 the need to observe the enemy meant that heads raised above the trench parapet became targets for sniper fire. High-velocity rifle bullets caused horrifying wounds to the face and jaw on a scale never seen before. The treatment of these injuries led to the emergence of a new branch of surgery – maxillo-facial surgery. A dentist pioneered this work, and today dentists carry a great share of the responsibility for maxillo-facial treatment. It must be remembered that treatment in the early days was done without benefit of sulphonamides and antibiotics. In the Great War, wounds were grossly contaminated with mud and bacteria. The relative slowness of casualty evacuation meant that gangrene was a constant problem.

The pioneer was Auguste Charles Valadier.

This remarkable man was born in Paris in 1873. His family emigrated to the United States in 1876 and Valadier became a naturalised American citizen. He qualified as a dentist at the Philadelphia Dental College in 1901. After working in New York, he returned to Paris in 1910 and practised there until the outbreak of the war in 1914. Valadier then offered his services to the British Red Cross. He was sent on duty to Abbeville in October 1914. Soon after, when dentists were first commissioned into the British Army, he was appointed as an honorary lieutenant on the General List.

The first individual to receive any official recognition by the War Office to treat injuries of the jaw was Charles Augustus Valadier, the American son of French parents who had practised in Paris. When war broke out, Valadier was practising at Place Vendome. He chose not to serve with the French because they did not have an organised dental corps at the time and dental care for their soldiers was provided in a very haphazard manner. Also, due to his age (forty years) and citizenship (United States), he was faced with the choice as a private in the French Army or service in the Foreign Legion. Given these choices, it is no wonder that Charles preferred to serve with the British.

Valadier volunteered his services to the British Red Cross Society and was dispatched in September to Abbeville, about a hundred miles north of Paris. From there he travelled another fifty miles until he found the British setting up a field headquarters around the port of Boulogne. Valadier was attached to the RAMC there and assigned to Number Thirteen General Hospital, which had just arrived from England on 16th October, 1914.

It is important to consider that the British Expeditionary Force had hurriedly deployed to France and the Low Countries without attaching a single dentist to provide for ninety thousand troops. Although the services of civilian dentists had been contracted since the Boer War, the British Army would not have a separate commissioned corps until 1921. So Valadier stepped into a vacuum on October 29th when he was accepted for duty with the British Forces in France. You can imagine how he impressed the British recruiting officers as he arrived at their headquarters in a chauffeur-driven Rolls-Royce. He was given the rank of 'Local Lieutenant', and attached to the RAMC at Boulogne.

During the same month, records indicate that Sir Douglas Haig, commanding the First Army about seventy miles north-east of Paris, was suffering from a severe toothache during the Battle of the Aisne. When it was discovered that a dental surgeon from Paris had to be summoned to provide a remedy for Haig's suffering, British authorities hurriedly requested that a dozen dentists be dispatched to serve the War Office in France. By the time they arrived early in November, Valadier had already been attached to the RAMC, thereby establishing himself as the first dentist to officially serve with the British Forces.

One cannot positively conclude that the 'dental surgeon from Paris' who treated General Haig was, in fact, Valadier. But the claim seems most plausible. For, if Valadier left Paris for Abbeville in September as reported, he would have been at or near the British General Headquarters during the Battle of the Aisne, coupled with the fact that Haig later recommended Valadier for a decoration in 1916:

> ...I cannot speak too highly of the excellent and most valuable surgical work on the jaw performed gratuitously by this gentleman for all ranks of the

British Army. He has performed a large number of operations on the jaws that require a high degree of surgical skill, with the most excellent results and which had not hitherto been attempted by the profession. I strongly recommend that he be given some tangible recognition of his services...

(*Signed*) D. Haig, General
April 30, 1916

This citation helped him obtain a temporary and honorary commission in the RAMC.

Early in 1915 he established a fifty bed unit attached to the Eighty-Third (Dublin) General Hospital at Wimereux near Boulogne for the treatment of facial injuries, bearing most of the cost of the organisation himself. Among his associates was Harold Gillies, who later established himself as one of the finest plastic surgeons of his time. His description of Valadier, published in 1957, reveals a remarkable picture:

> ...In Boulogne there was a great fat man with sandy hair and a florid face, who had equipped his Rolls-Royce with dental chair, drills and the necessary heavy metals. The name of this man, whose high riding boots carried a polish equal to the glitter of his spurs, was Charles Valadier. He toured about until he had filled with gold all the remaining teeth in British GHQ. With the generals strapped in his chair, he convinced them of the need of a plastic and jaw unit... the credit for establishing it, which so facilitated the later progress of plastic surgery, must go to the remarkable linguistic talents of the smooth and genial Sir Charles Valadier...

In addition to his Rolls-Royce dental operatory, Valadier also provided the equipment and laboratory technicians for the hospital unit at Wimereux. Most of the funds had come from earnings derived from his wealthy practice in Paris. Also, Valadier's widowed mother passed away in 1915, leaving him a considerable estate.

Valadier was granted a temporary and honorary rank of Major in the RAMC on April 30th, 1916. In 1918 he failed to reach the rank of Lieutenant Colonel, although he was well recommended for the promotion.

By January 1917 Valadier and his staff had treated more than one thousand cases of jaw and facial injuries. Many of the patients arrived in a septic and fetid state, two or three days after being wounded. Yet, in spite of the conditions, only twenty-seven deaths occurred – seven of these men were deemed beyond saving upon arrival.

Without doubt, Valadier was a skilled, resourceful and innovative oral surgeon. He was instrumental in both advancing and documenting improvements in maxillo-facial surgery during World War One.

A list of Valadier's awards and decorations includes the Companion of Saint Michael and Saint George (1916), Associate of Saint John of Jerusalem (1917), Chevalier of the Legion of Honour of France (1919), and finally Knight Commander of the Order of the British Empire (1919).

The only other dentist to be knighted for service during World War One was Sir Frank Colyer, whose base of operations was in England. Interestingly, Colyer and Valadier were bitter antagonists, as the methods of treatment advocated by each were sometimes diametrically opposed. Colyer eventually cared for many of the patients evacuated from Wimereux to the Croydon Jaw Hospital near London. He sometimes removed splints, extracted questionable teeth, and treated the inevitable sepsis which plagued all practitioners prior to the advent of penicillin. Valadier's methods, he claimed, were unsound.

After a chequered post war career, including a high run of gambling debts, Valadier died penniless, with a blood disease (possibly leukaemia), on August 31st 1931 at his villa in Le Touquet on the coast of Normandy.

MR WALKER JOINS THE GREAT WAR

[Lieut-Colonel G. V. Walker, RADC]

Soon after the 1914-1918 war commenced, the staff of the Newcastle-Upon-Tyne Dental Hospital offered free services to the Tyneside Scottish and Irish Brigades.

I was the senior student on extraction duty in the month of November and I extracted over nine hundred teeth in the month.

The men were extremely good patients. In those days we were only allowed to give two syringefuls of a solution of cocaine at one sitting. I remember a soldier who had all the uppers extracted and then said, "Now, what about the lowers?" I explained to him that I could not inject any more local anaesthetic, and so he said, "I'll have them out with nowt, as I want to get out to the front." Of course, we carried out other types of treatment in addition to extractions.

After qualifying, I went to assist a dental surgeon in Northallerton and there we had a very long day. At least half of our patients were in khaki and included a battalion of the Green Howards. Frequently, urgent calls were made for impressions in the morning and dentures to be fitted at evening. I believe that a number of our patients were seasick and some of our dentures went into the Channel. The Infantry Battalion was moved to Redcar in Yorkshire, and two days a week the boss and I chugged up in the old Ford car and visited the Coatham Convalescent Home. There we functioned in the saddleroom: two Windsor chairs back to back, the head on the knee, and performed operations there.

I had applied to the War Office for a commission as a dental surgeon immediately after qualifying, but was informed that there were five hundred candidates on the waiting list.

Eventually I had to join the ranks and went to the Royal Naval Division, serving at Cambrai, Passchendaele and the March Battle of

1918. My commission came through on March 22nd, but as we were in the firing line I was not allowed to move until April 27th, reaching Twenty-Three Casualty Clearing Station (CCS) on April 29th, where enormous numbers of patients turned up for treatment.

I had a very loyal clerk assistant, who wore thick spectacles and was knock-kneed. He lined up the patients, like an officer taking a parade, looked each from head to toe and said, "Have you been through the chair?"

The surgery was a place made of hessian canvas and poles, and the remarks of the patients could be plainly heard. I had a patient for an extraction and had to talk strongly to him to hold him to the point – fortunately the teeth came out clean without any pain. But my friend didn't like the 'strong' talking. A patient rolled up and said, "What's the dentist like?"

My friend said, "He's a funny sort of fellow, but he's all right." I am very proud of that, as the Tommy just summed me up correctly.

There were four divisions sending cases to the CCS. Three divisions had two days a week, but the First Division only had Sundays. Here I first met Claude G. Collier, who was in an advisory position to the First Army. He informed me that when I had seen thirty cases a day I could lay off – but of course I found this impossible.

Dentures were a constant source of trouble, as patients reported with all the sharp edges rounded off the broken ones, having carried them in their pockets for some time, necessitating remodelling. The laboratory would periodically shut down, and a sign be put up saying: NO MORE DENTURE CASES UNTIL FURTHER NOTICE.

I was posted to Thirty-Three Casualty Clearing Station at Douai, but here a bad attack of pneumonia kept me down and I was lucky to survive, as so many died in that epidemic of 1918.

Later I was sent to Osborne House and had forty very pleasant days there. After this I was posted to Cannock Chase, where we held a nice mixed Mess: three DOS, one MO, one RC Padre and an RASC Officer, Captain D. I. Isaac, with his pipe and a quiet sense of humour, who in spite of his one eye was a great help in the Mess.

The surgeries were upstairs and the waiting-room also. One morning as we passed through the patients, a voice was heard to say, "The little b*****d is the best."

After this I had a short spell at Catterick Garrison where I was bombed. Then I went to take charge of the practice at Northallerton, the 'boss' being ill.

Fortunately he soon recovered and the War Office offered new terms for officers going out to India. I rejoined. It was a twelve month contract with a possibility of renewal. I was posted to Tidworth prior to embarkation and arrived in India in May 1920.

WORLD WAR II – DUNKIRK – MISSING BELIEVED KILLED

Colonel F. J. W. Hooper, RAMC (Rtd) cast his mind back thirty years to recall the events of that time. He wrote as follows:

I was Regimental Medical Officer to the Second Battalion Lancashire Fusiliers in Eleven Infantry Brigade and belonging to Four Division during the retreat to Dunkirk, and during the sea evacuation of the British Expeditionary Force (BEF) in May and June 1940.

In the early morning of 1st June 1940, the battalion was called forward for sea evacuation from the makeshift piers in front of the town of Oostdunkirk, on the extreme left of the beach head. During embarkation, the German artillery put down a barrage on the piers, scattering those personnel who had not already embarked. At dawn, the battalion medical orderly (L/Cpl Knowles) a stretcher bearer (Fusilier Wasserman) and I were walking along the beach, when we met the Brigade Commander and his Brigade Major, and we were instructed to proceed along the beach to the town of Dunkirk. About a mile further on, I observed the dental officer and padre of Eleven Field Ambulance in a shell hole. The shell hole was level with the outskirts of the town of Oostdunkirk and about fifty yards from the water's edge. My party then sat down in the shell hole, and we all discussed the situation and our plans. The dental officer and padre stated that they intended to join a queue of officers and soldiers that was already stretching into the shallows awaiting sea transport. I informed these officers that my party was proceeding along the beach in the direction of the town of Dunkirk. We then parted.

It would seem a reasonable assumption that the dental officer and padre did join the column of BEF personnel in the shallow water, and subsequently they were either (a) machine gunned from the air in the shallow water or (b) they embarked on a ship, and the ship was sunk off shore by dive bombers.

About six weeks after my party arrived in England, a circular letter was issued by HQ Four Division asking for information concerning missing personnel and I think a list of names was appended. I am almost certain that I sent in a statement concerning my meeting with the dental officer and padre of Eleven Infantry Brigade on the lines as stated above.

It eventually transpired that Jameson and his padre companion both died as a result of being machine gunned, while awaiting evacuation.

A DENTAL OFFICER DEPARTS DUNKIRK, MAY 1940

[Colonel J.E Maywhort, Late Royal Army Dental Corps]

I was attached to Thirteen Field Ambulance as a Captain in the Army Dental Corps. We mobilised in York and moved to France. We were stationed in Biach, St Vaast, when we got our orders to pull back to Dunkirk where we were meant to open operations.

I do not remember much about the move, the weather was fine and there was quite a lot of aerial activity. A few pilots were bailing out, with shouts from the French civilians, "Parachutist," and shots from the ground. Our stretcher bearer brought in an RAF pilot. He was dead on arrival at the dressing station, the surgeon traced the bullet, and it had definitely come from below.

We arrived uneventfully at Dunkirk and we were told to abandon our vehicles and get on the boats moored at the quayside. I got on a Dutch canal boat with Royal Navy Crew, the O/ic hoped that my Red Cross armband would not be needed. He said I could not use his sleeping cabin as two French girls were in there!

He gave me a drink, clear liquid. I thought it was water, knocked it back – it was gin. I slept halfway across on the floor of his day cabin, it was a clear sunny day – no trouble. We disembarked at Ramsgate or Margate.

On the train I asked a Guards Officer (RTO) if I could send a telegram, he gave me a sheet of paper for my wife's address and the message. He sent it off and my wife received it.

I cannot remember much after that. The field ambulance reformed at Southwell. I do not think we had any casualties.

D-DAY 1944 – OPERATIONAL DENTISTS DROP IN

The dental personnel of the Parachute Field Ambulances of 6 Airborne Division (Nos 195, 224, and 225) dropped with their field ambulances on the night of 5/6 June 1944, emergency dental treatment being available on 6th June 1944 with the equipment carried in the dental haversacks. Full field dental equipment was later supplied to them by the issue of panniers from Advanced Depot Medical Stores reserves.

The dental personnel of the field ambulances of the assaulting formations (Three (BR) Division and Fifty (N) Division) landed on D-Day, as did the dental personnel of Five, Seven and Eight Beach Group Field Dressing Stations (i.e. One, Two, Twenty, Thirty-Three and Thirty-Four Field Dressing Stations), Thirty-One Field Dressing Station (Ten Beach Group), and Thirty-Five Field Dressing Station (Nine Beach Group). The arrival of the dental officers of Ten Casualty Clearing Station (Thirty Corps) and Sixteen and Seventeen Field Dressing Stations (Forty-nine Division) brought the total number of dental officers present in Normandy on the evening of D-Day to twenty, a proportion of one dental officer to three thousand men.

In all cases, until the arrival of their full equipment (in most cases a matter of a few days), dental officers of the assault units were restricted to the provision of emergency dental treatment only. In addition to these duties, they assisted the medical units by the performance of minor operations and the administration of anaesthetics; services much valued by the officers commanding medical units.

DENTAL OFFICERS INVOLVED IN THE NORMANDY LANDINGS (D-DAY), 1944

Dental Officers involved in the Normandy Landings

Unit	Officer	Date
9 Gen Hosp	G Armytage	10 Jul 44
74 Gen Hosp	P Cummings	09 Jul 44
77 Gen Hosp	H V Newcombe	22 Jun 44
81 Gen Hosp	E H Bird	10 Jun 44
84 Gen Hosp	O C Thomson	17 Jun 44
86 Gen Hosp	HDP Hughes	10 Jun 44
88 Gen Hosp	A Baker	22 Jun 44
121 Gen Hosp	A R Ferguson	12 Jul 44
79 Gen Hosp	G M Kindness	16 Jun 44
3 CGS	E B Cheffins	07 Jun 44
10 CGS	G B Ashworth	06 Jun 44
16 CGS	J F Blenkinsop	14 Jun 44
23 CGS	GJM Hughes	26 Jul 44
24 CGS	L A Sewell	26 Jul 44
32 CGS	B G Wood	12 Jun 44
33 CGS	J O Sykes	30 Jun 44
34 CGS	W L Trick	26 Jun 44
35 CGS	A J Boylin	11 Jun 44
1 FDS	F J Summers	06 Jun 44
2 FDS	A Blair	06 Jun 44
3 FDS	F A Soper	12 Jun 44
4 FDS	T L White	26 Jul 44
5 FDS	W C Arkle	02 Jul 44
6 FDS	G U Lyle	02 Jul 44
7 FDS	R S Henderson	15 Jun 44
8 FDS	E W Wright	15 Jul 44
9 FDS	K Howse	26 Jul 44
10 FDS	J L Deuchar	10 Jun 44
11 FDS	JET Morris	12 Jun 44
12 FDS	J McN Richardson	26 Jul 44
13 FDS	J M Millett	27 Jun 44
14 FDS	FJC Hood	13 Jun 44
15 FDS	S F Fish	13 Jul 44
16 FDS	E A Haxton	06 Jun 44
17 FDS	S Ford	06 Jun 44
20 FDS	ETJ Dykes	06 Jun 44
21 FDS	W F Dunn	06 Jun 44
22 FDS	RGD Gordon	23 Jun 44
23 FDS	F Parkinson	12 Jul 44
25 FDS	J F Briscoe	19 Jul 44
26 FDS	G B Crichton	27 Jun 44
26 FDS	J Cranfield	26 Jul 44
28 FDS	A W Donald	26 Jul 44
29 FDS	E P Cutler	12 Jun 44
30 FDS	C A Cuthbertson	25 Jun 44
31 FDS	D E Ashdown	06 Jun 44
32 FDS	IDM Jones	26 Jul 44
33 FDS	D H Bowman	06 Jun 44
34 FDS	P K Hopkins	06 Jun 44
35 FDS	J Redgate	06 Jun 44
47 FDS	G G Mowatt	13 Jun 44
48 FDS	J K Lindsay	13 Jun 44
49 FDS	H T Mason	08 Jun 44
50 FDS	M J Camber	15 Jun 44
147 FDC	F Stephenson	24 Jul 44
147 FDC	D A Ward	24 Jul 44
13 Con Dep	F W Sander	12 Jul 44
500 Mob D U	W J Duval	22 Jun 44
501 Mob D U	CGW Harrison	24 Jun 44
502 Mob D U	D D Stalford	16 Jun 44
503 Mob D U	G R Gilberg	21 Jun 44
504 Mob D U	A H Herbert	22 Jun 44
505 Mob D U	R W Marston	22 Jun 44
506 Mob D U	E A Meadows	24 Jun 44
507 Mob D U	A D Dunlop	25 Jun 44
508 Mob D U	D M Martyn	24 Jun 44
509 Mob D U	G R Atkins	19 Jun 44
510 Mob D U	C S Syms	24 Jun 44
511 Mob D U	A Kinghorn	24 Jun 44
512 Mob D U	JRL Toleman	14 Jul 44
515 Mob D U	JKB Salmond	27 Jun 44
8 Fd Amb	F E Street	06 Jun 44
9 Fd Amb	J L Hutton	06 Jun 44
128 Fd Amb	E H C-Clark	15 Jul 44
129 Fd Amb	G H English	15 Jun 44
130 Fd Amb	H W Abson	19 Jun 44
131 Fd Amb	R Stanley	12 Jun 44
146 Fd Amb	J E Roberts	10 Jun 44
147 Fd Amb	J A Pilling	23 Jun 44
149 Fd Amb	G D Fleetwood	06 Jun 44
153 Fd Amb	F Edwards	28 Jun 44
160 Fd Amb	J H Humphreys	11 Jun 44
174 Fd Amb	B Hirschfield	07 Jun 44
175 Fd Amb	G H Guest	08 Jun 44
176 Fd Amb	A F Campbell	11 Jun 44
179 Fd Amb	JEH Bell	05 Jul 44
186 Fd Amb	G Pascall	06 Jun 44
187 Fd Amb	E R Hanlan	13 Jun 44
193 Fd Amb	K A Keith	18 Jun 44
194 Fd Amb	T D Grandison	22 Jun 44
200 FD Amb	R McCleod	06 Jun 44
202 Fd Amb	P C Hallsworth	27 Jun 44
203 Fd Amb	NBH McGrath	26 Jun 44
210 Fd Amb	L E Donaldson	26 Jun 44
211 Fd Amb	R E Savage	26 Jun 44
212 Fd Amb	J K Whitelaw	27 Jun 44
214 Fd Amb	A Hay	24 Jun 44
223 Fd Amb	J P Blunt	06 Jun 44
2 Lt Fd Amb	P B Reid	10 Jul 44
11 Lt Fd Amb	FSS Brooks	12 Jul 44
14 Lt Fd Amb	A Fraser	15 Jun 44
16 Lt Fd Amb	EGW Lewis	25 Jun 44
18 Lt Fd Amb	H L Saunders	05 Jul 44
19 Lt Fd Amb	E L Evans	28 Jun 44
21 Lt Fd Amb	RKP Miller	16 Jun 44
22 Lt Fd Amb	WFA Butcher	18 Jun 44
23 Lt Fd Amb	D A Miller	18 Jun 44
168 Lt Fd Amb	I C Brown	13 Jun 44
194 AB Fd Amb	Holland	
224 AB Fd Amb	Chaundy	
225 AB Fd Amb	A N Other	

The conduct and bearing of dental officers in the assault received much praise from their commanding officers. Some dental officers, upon whom the sole charge of personnel in assault boats had devolved, showed the most commendable courage, initiative, and leadership in landing their charges and equipment in the face of intense enemy fire. The hazards of the operation were greatly increased by the heavy seas then running, the presence of uncleared underwater obstacles, and obstructions caused by boats and ships which had become derelict or had broached to. For his conduct on this day the dental officer of Eight Field Ambulance (Capt. F. A. Street) received the immediate award of the Military Cross.

When landing on D+15, the vehicle of 209 Mobile Dental Unit (Capt. E. R. Meadows), was 'drowned' in four foot six inches of water. It was dried out and made serviceable in two days, personnel and equipment having suffered no mishap or damage.

During the actions continuously fought to expand the bridgehead, the dental personnel of medical units accompanied them in all operations; their regimental value, particularly as advanced party recce officers for laagers, were highly spoken of by officers commanding units.

Due to the frequent movement of their units, dental officers of field ambulances and Field Dressing Stations were able to open for dental treatment for only fourteen days a month on average during June and July. The output of professional work was considered good, bearing in mind the difficulties under which it was performed. A time lag of about a day occurred on the arrival of a dental officer in a locality before the neighbouring units became aware of its presence. Quiescent periods, so called, were times reduced by infantry combat during which harassing action from artillery, mortar and small arms fire and from air continued (and was frequently intensified) on rearward divisional targets.

It was during such times that the dental officer of 211 Field Ambulance (Fifty-nine Division), Capt. R. E. Savage, was killed by enemy air attack and the dental officer of Six Field Dressing Station (Forty-one (H) Division), Capt. C. U. Lyle was wounded. In such circumstances, it was not unusual for patients to request the postponement of dental treatment.

The dental personnel of divisional Mobile Dental Units worked under the same conditions as those attached to Medical Units, being sited in most cases about two to three miles behind the troops actively engaged. Owing to their independence of action, they were able to remain open for longer periods, averaging about twenty-four days a month. Though no casualties to personnel were experienced by Mobile Dental Units, the shelters number fourteen (penthouses) of three vehicles were damaged by shell or bomb fragments, the exhaust silencer of one being severed by the 'air burst' of an eighty-eight millimetre shell.

The enthusiasm of Mobile Dental unit personnel in executing the 'forward of treatment' policy was such that it became necessary to recall 209 Mobile Dental unit (Guards Armoured Division) Capt. E. S. Meadows from the night laager[1] of a squadron of the RAC, situated in the neighbourhood of Cuverville (MR105690). The engagement leading to the clearing of Caen and the armoured advance to Bourgebus was imminent, and the laager was under heavy fire on the night of 17/18th July 1944.

During the preceding night, 210 Mobile Dental Unit (Eleven Armoured Division) Capt. A. D. Dunlop was observed to have taken up a position between two tank squadrons in the column of route during the lateral move of the armoured divisions across the front to concentrate East of Caen.

Intimate association in this manner with the units under their care was only possible by the removal of the Geneva emblem from their vehicles, carried out under instructions issued in the UK.

Second Army – Final Phase

During the Battle of Falaise – and subsequently until a slight pause on the Meuse-Escaut Canal – contact with dental officers of formations became increasingly difficult. Dental officers made their professional services available at every opportunity offered by short halts between periods of movement.

The value of specialist vehicles in providing almost continuous treatment during moves was well demonstrated. The dental officers of 210 MDU (Captain A. D. Dunlop) of Eleven Armoured Division, 131 Fld Amb. (Capt. Stanley) and Two Light Fld Amb. (Capt. Reid), both of Seven Amrd Division, had each obtained through divisional admin. channels a three ton lorry converted by REME into a Mobile Dental Surgery. It was then possible to provide treatment even on brief roadside halts.

---

[1]   South African (Boers) term for a field position

The final phase of operations – the crossing of the Rhine and the advance to the Baltic – brought into it opportunities for the operational employment of dental units and personnel similar to those presented in Northern France and Belgium.

The dental personnel of Second Army were, with few exceptions, those who landed with it in Normandy and had taken part in all its actions with regimental and professional distinction.

Captain B. Hirschfield, Army Dental Corps, attached 174 Field Ambulance (31 Highland Div), was granted the immediate award of the Military Cross for his conduct in the opening stages of this final phase of operations.

AWARD OF THE MILITARY CROSS – CITATIONS AD CORPS

Captain B. Hirschfield MC, The Army Dental Corps (Rhine Crossing)

Knowing that the unit was short of medical officers, Captain Hirschfield, Dental Officer of 174 (H) Fd Amb., volunteered to take command of one of the two Casualty Evacuation Points which were to cross the river Rhine, on the night of 23rd/24th March 1945 with the assault troops of 153 Infantry Brigade.

With his section and carrying light medical equipment, he crossed the river at H+30 minutes and rapidly established his CEP on the East Bank at Map Ref. 055523, approximately one mile west of REES.

During the night, when his stock of stretchers and blankets for casualties were becoming exhausted, he recrossed the river in face of extremely troublesome shell and mortar fire on both banks and at the crossing site, contacted the officer i/c Cas Disembarkation Point and made sure that there would be no failure in replenishment of these and other medical stores.

Soon after his return to the CEP, a Bren carrier, which had just been disembarked from a LVT and was proceeding inland towards the vehicle assembling area, received a direct hit from a shell, about two hundred yards from the CEP. Despite the continued shelling and disregarding the danger of mines, Captain Hirschfield immediately ran out with a stretcher party to the wrecked carrier, rendered first aid to four badly wounded members of its crew and had them carried to the shelter and comparative safety of trenches dug in the vicinity of the CEP from which they were subsequently safely evacuated.

Bitter enemy resistance continued in REES until 25th March and from observation points in the town, the enemy were able frequently to direct accurate shell and mortar fire on the LVT crossing in the immediate neighbourhood of the CEP. Nevertheless, throughout the night of 23rd/24th March and during the two succeeding days Captain Hirschfield continued his work with the utmost determination.

His coolness, complete disregard for his own safety and his unfailing cheerfulness in all circumstances were undoubtably a fine example to all his men and contributed greatly to the success of the evacuation arrangements.

Captain F. E. Street, MC, AD Corps (D-Day Normandy)

This officer landed on Queen White Beach at H+60 minutes under heavy mortar and machine-gun fire.

On reaching the cover of some small sand dunes where an improvised dressing station had been organised by personnel of this unit, he formed stretcher parties to bring in casualties from the beaches. His coolness and determination under fire did a great deal to inspire confidence into the stretcher bearers who brought in a large number of casualties.

After the beach had been swept, he carried on working in the dressing station – again in a manner which inspired confidence in both orderlies and patients.

His conduct was more noticeable as this was the first landing Captain Street had made from any type of craft, and he was extremely seasick whilst on board.

DENTISTS AND WAR – A FILM IS MADE

"We made an educational film for surgeons that caused distress at Wembley. It had an awkward title – *Treatment of Maxillo-Facial Injuries in the Field* – but the content was memorable. Much of it was photographed in a forward area... Rhine crossings. Men, our own, and prisoners were brought in at the point of death with their jaws shot away... The filming was supervised by a Captain... James Dyce (Army Dental Corps).

The distress was mainly in the film cutting rooms. None of the senior editors could look at the material, even in a movieola, without being taken ill. I had difficulty and was tempted to make excuses for not seeing the rushes when they arrived from the lab. The only person, apart from Jimmy Dyce, who viewed them with enthusiasm was an ATS assistant cutter. In the end she took over the editing. She did an excellent job."

The two reels, each which runs for forty minutes, gives a vivid picture of the horrors and triumphs of the medical and dental services in Europe during World War Two. Copies went to all the principal medical and dental schools in the allied army.

From the Book *The Lies of Eric Ambler* (who in World War Two was a colonel in the army and a film director to the Army Kinematograph Service.)

TO INDIA and BURMA VIA THE MEDITERRANEAN – A WORLD WAR TWO ACCOUNT

[Major D. F. Glass, AD Corps]

The Fifth British Division was probably the most travelled division in the war, hence its name 'The Globe Trotters', and as the dental officer to the 164 Field Ambulance, thirteenth Brigade for more than four years, I am probably one of the widest travelled members of the Corps.

I joined the Fifth Division after its withdrawal from Dunkirk, when it reformed in Aberdeenshire. During the autumn of 1940 we moved to Lancashire and in January 1941 we moved to Northern Ireland, and along with two other divisions we sat on the Eire border ready to cross if Southern Ireland were invaded from Europe. At the end of 1942, we returned to England and Surrey where we were mobilised for the Far East. We sailed from the Clyde in Spring 1942 and eventually arrived in South Africa after a short call at Freetown in West Africa.

At this time, the Allied shipping was suffering heavily in the Mozambique Channel from Japanese submarines who were refuelling at Diego Suarez in the northern tip of Madagascar. On the 5th May 1942, the division took part in the assault landing, capturing Diego Suarez in four days.

After three weeks, we embarked for India where we started intensive training for the Burma front.

The war in Eastern Europe during the autumn of 1942 was causing much anxiety. Rommel was all powerful in North Africa, and the Germans had swept into Russia and had turned south between the Black Sea and the Caspian Sea and had almost reached the Caucasus Mountains.

The Fifth Division was ordered from India to Persia, where we prepared to hold a line north of Sennah in North Persia. We arrived in Persia in the autumn of 1942 and left in the spring of 1943 after a very cold and uncomfortable winter spent at an altitude between four thousand and six thousand feet.

With the recession of the threat to Persia, we turned west, crossing the vast Iraqi desert to the Mediterranean. Special intensive training was carried out in mountain warfare, and at the Cedars of Lebanon we learned the ways of the worthy mule to replace our ambulances in hilly country. At the Suez Canal we familiarised ourselves with the assault landing craft in preparation for the invasion of Europe.

On July 5th we embarked at Suez for Operation Husky and formed part of the Eastern Task Force to capture Sicily. D-Day was July 10th. I got ashore at H+11 and was well clear of the landing beach by the time the enemy bombers came in force. The Sicilian campaign was hot, dusty and exhausting, but after six weeks we were at rest on the side of Mount Etna, preparing for Operation Baytown, the assault landing on the mainland of Europe.

The landing in Italy across the Straits of Messina was the Division's third D-Day, and, being September 3rd, it was exactly four years after the outbreak of war.

The advance through Italy was slow and arduous. Orsona on the Adriatic Coast was reached by Christmas 1943 and represented an advance of three hundred and eighty miles in four months, to a position north of Rome but separated by the high Appenines.

In January 1944 we moved to the Casino front, the Division crossing the Garigliano river despite heavy opposition. In March we moved to the Anzio beach to relieve the exhausted fifty-sixth Division and by June 4th we were sitting on the bank by the Tiber River. Rome was captured at the same time as D-Day in North Europe, so we really felt we were getting on with the work.

The Fifth Division had been in continuous action for a year and was by now exhausted by fatigue and casualties. It is interesting that in the Anzio Beach Head alone, our casualties were a hundred and sixty officers and three thousand men. We withdrew from the line and returned to Egypt, Palestine and Syria to refit and train for Northern Europe.

In October 1944 I left the 164 Fd Amb. of the Fifth Division to join the Ninety-First General Hospital in Gaza. This was indeed a sad departure. I gave up my camp bed for a feather bed and my fighting friends for a bunch of 'Base Wallahs'. However, the war in Europe was nearly over and I was pleased to become a dental specialist with the rank of Major.

In retrospect, I had a most interesting war, if somewhat hazardous at times. I visited fourteen different countries and took part in three assault landings.

A BUSY CAREER
THROUGH FRANCE
[Colonel Matt Gemmell, Late RADC]

As a young officer I played both soccer and rugby with much pleasure, but without distinction. I played a fair game of tennis and at golf won the Corps Championship and the Society Cup.

At the start of World War Two, I mobilised with Number One Field Ambulance and went to France in September 1939 to care for the dental problems of the First Guards Brigade. There, while on the move through France by road, I extracted teeth for half a dozen soldiers on the grass verge at the roadside. Instruments were sterilised in a 'dixie', and boiled up on a primus stove borrowed from the cooks. The patients sat on a folding wooden chair, the headrest was provided by the chest of the dental orderly.

A month or so later, my dental sick parade was so large that between 0845 and 1315 hours one day I extracted ninety-six teeth, all under local anaesthesia, using the field chair and field equipment. The work at this time was not all extractions, many fillings being completed using the foot-treadle engine.

I did not get out of France until two weeks after the Dunkirk troops had been evacuated. The departure from France was facilitated by the 'acquisition' of a small French motor car in which I drove my Commanding Officer (RAMC) about 375 miles due west in two days, eventually getting out by ship from St Nazaire.

GREECE EXPEDITIONARY FORCE – THE DENTAL PRESENCE

Following the despatch of an expeditionary force to Greece, three additional dental officers arrived in the country at the beginning of March 1941, attached to British Medical Units allotted to the force. These units were Number Twenty-Four Casualty Clearing Station, Number Four and Number 168 Light Field Ambulances.

Before the German invasion, Number Twenty-Six General Hospital was located near Athens; Number Twenty-Four Casualty Clearing Station at Larissa; and Number 168 Field Amb. in the Edepa Area Number Four Light Field Ambulance was with Number One Armoured Brigade.

All these units had dental personnel attached. As a result of the German invasion and their attack on Greece, the majority of the medical units were successfully evacuated and disembarked in Crete. They brought with them no transport and virtually no equipment. The total number of dental officers in Crete before the German Airborne Invasion was ten – four British Army, two Royal Navy, two New Zealand, and two Australian Forces. There were six dental mechanics – three British and three New Zealand. Seven dental clerk orderlies, of whom four were British, two New Zealand, and one Australian.

It was only possible to do emergency extractions and temporary fillings for the troops who attended for treatment. Two British dental officers were attached to Number Seven General Hospital and they were assisted by the dental officers of Number Five New Zealand Field Ambulance. The laboratory equipment at this hospital was shared by four dental mechanics. Some dental work was undertaken by a local private dental practitioner on a very limited scale.

Number Seven General Hospital was captured by German parachutists during the first few hours of the attack. Three officers of the Army Dental Corps were taken prisoner. The New Zealand Dental Services were mainly despatched in numbers as a result of the operations in Greece and Crete.

Captain Cook (New Zealand Dental Corps) volunteered to help Captain Cooper, the British Army dental officer who had arrived with remnants of the Number Twenty-Six (Br) General Hospital from Greece. Captain Cook was later captured, and he was later to join Captain K. C. Blanthorne, the Army Dental Corps in captivity in Poland. The New Zealanders took a philosophical view of the capture of so many dental officers, orderlies and mechanics; they were a boon to their fellow prisoners of war.

ANOTHER WORLD WAR TWO TRUE STORY FROM A NARVIK AND SEABORNE TA RESERVE DO

[Bertram Bland, Retired general practitioner, Honorary Dental Surgeon, West Suffolk General Hospital]

Robert Cutler's interesting wartime true story (*British Dental Journal*, October 2, 1979) prompts me to respond with a personal wartime experience which certainly taught me to 'Judge not that ye be not judged'. Having a non-active dental officer's commission in the TA Reserve, I was mobilised on September 2nd, 1939, and by April/May 1940 I found myself serving with a field ambulance in the Norwegian Narvik Sector.

In the town of Harstad on the Lofoten Islands, one G. B. Drury, dental officer of the military hospital, had taken over the surgery of a Norwegian dentist who was serving in their forces, and so had his own field dental outfit spare. I spent most of my time using it alongside him, doing our best to cope with the desperate dental needs and neglect of the ex-civilians, mobilised into the Armed Forces.

Our army had the enemy ground troops under control in the Narvik sector, but some two hundred miles to the south, near Bodo, the Scots Guards were in real trouble, so higher command sent a battalion of Irish Guards, with a company liner Chrobury, to back them up. Jerry, who virtually had complete air superiority, dropped a bomb on the liner, which exploded in the stateroom where officers were in conference and that was that.

To prevent a repetition of this tragedy, a battalion of South Wales Borderers and our HQ Coy of the 137 Field Ambulance were crammed on to the anti-aircraft cruiser HMS *Effingham* which, together with another ack-ack cruiser, HMS *Coventry* and two destroyers, set out a few days later for Bodo.

One of the first things I did was to offer my services to the Principal Medical Officer (PMO) aboard, who was delighted as the cruiser had undergone a £3 million refit and come straight to Norwegian waters from a six month shakedown cruise in the West Indies. This meant that the crew had not been near a naval dental centre for a long time.

There was no dental chair in the sick bay, so the ship's carpenter, or chippy, fixed a broomhead covered with a towel to the high back of the admiral's chair. Short crew members had to sit bolt upright and tall ones slid down of course, but it served its purpose well. When, with the ship's forceps and syringes, we were all set to go. The message went out over the tannoy that there was an 'army toothwright' aboard and anyone who had toothache and had had toothache or thought they might get toothache was to report to the sick bay or forever hold their peace.

They started with a trickle which became a stream and (perhaps as they got back to their stations and said it didn't hurt) the stream grew into a flood. I worked all day with no more than a couple of breaks for coffee and sandwiches. Many of the ratings had fortified themselves liberally with rum for the ordeal and that tiny sickbay soon stank of it.

Outside in the companionway, some boosted their ego with loud and bawdy ribaldry and this, my first encounter with the 'lower deck' *en masse*, did not exactly fill me with admiration and respect for them.

As the last patient left, one Surgeon Lieutenant Excel rushed me to the wardroom for a much-needed meal because, he explained, we were already sailing up the Bodo fiord and would be disembarking in an hour or so. With so many army officers in excess of the normal ship's complement, there was not a seat to be had, so he instructed a steward to call us immediately. One was available and he took me up on the gun deck for a breath of fresh air.

What a glorious sight met our eyes. It was approaching the time of the midnight sun, and although it was evening the sun was still high in a cloudless, blue sky. We were belting up the fiord at about twenty-three knots, with snow-clad mountains on either side, ending in a black line where the sea had washed the snow off the rock. Ahead of us the foaming wake of the destroyer HMS *Echo* and half a mile astern the giant bow wave of the *Coventry*. I was spellbound for about two minutes and then... she struck! Four feet or so of uncharted rock over which she ground her way, ripping her bottom out, and wallowed into deeper water on the other side. The *Echo* rushed back to us and tied up forrard. The discipline and efficiency of both crews was magnificent, and within about quarter of an hour (by which time the *Effingham*'s quarter-deck was awash) they had somehow crammed about eight hundred troops and five hundred of the seven hundred and fifty crew on to, and into, that tiny destroyer.

When not another man could be squeezed on to the *Echo*, we cast off, leaving some two hundred and fifty of those grand chaps in their lifejackets lining the *Effingham*'s upper decks. We knew, and they knew, that no one could survive more than a couple of minutes in those waters north of the Arctic Circle and yet, as we pulled away, they gave us a cheer! My heart and my eyes filled as I realised that these were the men for whom earlier that day I had felt some contempt.

The *Echo* shipped us on to the *Coventry*, which took us back to Harstad. Some days later I learnt to my great relief that, while taking us aboard, the *Echo* had been pushing the *Effingham* back towards the reef and she had actually grounded long enough for the rest of the crew to be saved.

There was an amusing aftermath, when at Harstad we were ferried to the shore launches. From the stern of one of these I saw a middle-aged rating up in the bows look furtively around to see if anyone was looking, then put his hand over his mouth and thence over the side. I did not then know that dentures lost through shipwreck may be replaced without question.

The next day I was again working alongside G. B. Drury, and one of the first patients I saw was this rating with a note from a naval MO requesting the replacement of full dentures lost in shipwreck. To his horror, I was able to tell him exactly where and how he had lost them, but then I reassured him by saying that after what they had done for us there was nothing I would not do for them. He explained that he had had dentures for about a year and they had given him hell from the day he got them. With the excellent prosthetics facilities available at the military hospital I was glad to fix him up in a matter of days.

AN AIRBORNE DENTAL SERVICE

[Edited extract from the Book *On Wings of Healing* by
Howard N. Cole, OBE., TD., FRHistS]

The 127th Parachute Field Ambulance (PFA) took part in Operation Anvil, the invasion of Southern France, the dental officer being Captain Brown, AD Corps.

D-Day, the invasion of Normandy, took place on the night of 5th/6th June 1944, and was code named OPERATION OVERLORD. Capt. C. A. Chaundy, AD Corps reported together with three other ranks to the Medical Dressing Station at Les Mesnil just after midday. This was part of the 224th PFA. Medical cover was given during the first seventy-seven days after the invasion, until the Sixth Airborne Division was withdrawn to the United Kingdom for further training.

On the 17th/18th of September 1944, the airborne landing at Arnhem took place, the object of which was to take and hold the bridge in advance of the Second Army. The Sixteenth and 133rd PFA and the 181st Fd Amb. formed the medical cover to the 1st British Airborne Division. By 2130 hours on 17th September, the Sixteenth PFA had reached St Elizabeth Hospital, situated in the western part of Arnhem. At 0800 hours, on Monday 18th September, after heavy firing, German troops moved past the hospital, which was then recaptured. The Wehrmach agreed that two surgical teams – comprising two surgeons, two anaesthetists, one of whom was Capt. D. H. Ridler MC, and fifteen other ranks – could remain in the hospital, the remainder of the Sixteenth PFA were marched away as prisoners of war.

Soon SS Troops occupied the hospital and even placed a guard on the operating theatre door. They soon left, after seeing a particularly unpleasant amputation in front of them.

Meanwhile, fighting was becoming heavy and confused. The GOC, returning from scenes of house fighting to Divisional Headquarters, told the Assistant Director of Medical Services (ADMS), Colonel S. M. Warrack, that Sixteenth PFA was hard at work in the St Elizabeth Hospital and that it might be possible to contact them by telephone.

This was achieved, the telephone being answered by the Dental Officer, Capt. D. H. Ridler MC, who told the ADMS that he was standing in a booth by the main entrance to the hospital "and it was rather difficult to hear". This was to be one of the understatements of the day, for there was in fact a pitched battle going on in and around the grounds, the conversation being punctuated by the crash of shell fire and the rattle of machine guns just outside. Capt. Ridler was able to give the ADMS a good picture of the position – he had been left with surgical teams, about twenty all ranks to deal with almost one hundred casualties.

The conversation ended with a loud explosion and an assurance from Capt. Ridler "that the detachment was in good heart".

By early Wednesday 20th September all that was left of the 133rd PFA were the CO, his two surgeons, the Dental Officer Capt. A. S. Flockhart AD Corps, and one hundred other ranks. They were captured at Oosterbeek, their operating theatre, a Dutch dentist's surgery, being deliberately wrecked by a small party of German infantrymen.

Communication between the DZs was hazardous. All ranks RAMC carried Red Cross flags when they moved about. Food was becoming short. Capt. P. Griffin AD Corps, the Dental Officer of the 181st AL Fd Amb, killed two sheep with a Sten gun. These were made into stew.

On the 25th September, Capt. Griffin was sent to supervise the evacuation of a Regimental Aid Post (RAP), the MO being wounded. He went down to the river and brought back about twenty wounded lying there.

Under cover of a barrage that night, the withdrawal took place. The Medical Services stayed behind to help those who would shortly become prisoners of war.

Soon, the wounded selected by the MO were paraded and searched, given a cup of tea and a blanket. Three Medical Officers and the Dental Officer – Capt. D. H. Ridler – were detailed to entrain. These four officers had been assured that they would be permitted to tend to the wounded. They were in fact locked into their carriages. Under these circumstances they decided to try and escape. They drew lots to see who should remain, as they felt that one of them should. Capt. Simmons RAMC stayed. The other three jumped the train. In the escape, Capt. Keesay RAMC was shot dead by a guard, but Capt. Ridler and Capt. Lawson got clean away in the darkness and successfully escaped.

Crossing the Rhine took place on the morning of 24 March 1945, (Operation Varsity). Units of the Sixth Airborne Division landed just south of Dierfordterwald. The DZ for the 224th PFA was a wooded area and a number of the unit landed in high trees – three were killed in the drop, one being the padre. The other personnel disentangled themselves and made for the rendezvous. As they neared the position, Capt. C. A. Chaundy, the Dental Officer, was shot through the neck and died instantly.

During the advance to the Baltic, 244th PFA arrived at Wissenden, during an engagement with the enemy, Capt. Naysmith, the Dental Officer, was taken prisoner while putting up directional signs to the Medical Dressing Station. However, by the afternoon he had been liberated by the Royal Ulster Rifles. Capt. Naysmith had tried his best to persuade a German company commander to surrender, but without avail. His stubbornness resulted in few prisoners being taken that day by the RUR, who laid a trail of smoke and fire from farms and buildings, as well as leaving many German dead.

On the morning of May 7th, all German Armies in Europe surrendered. Soon afterwards, having first served in Norway, the Sixteenth AL Fd Amb. was disbanded at Perham Down, near Tidworth.

The Sixtieth and Eightieth (Indian) and the Seventh (British) PFAs saw service in the Far East, as did 225th PFA. The atomic bombs dropped on Hiroshima and Nagasaki brought about the capitulation of Japan.

The 127th and 224th PFA and the 195th AL Fd Amb. served in Palestine between 1945 and 1948.

The 127th PFA was reformed. It was originally the 127th (East Lancashire) Field Ambulance RAMC (TA). It was given the regular army number of the Twenty-third PFA.

The Sixth Airborne Division was disbanded in the summer of 1948, the Regular Airborne Forces being reduced to a single brigade group. The Second Parachute Brigade was selected to become the permanent airborne element of the regular army. It was renumbered and redesignated the Sixteenth Independent Parachute Brigade Group. This consisted of the First, Second, and Third Battalions of the Parachute Regiment. The Twenty-Third PFA became part of this brigade.

In June 1951 the Twenty-Third PFA embarked for Cyprus and on the 18th October landed at Suez, where it remained until 1954. A section returned to Cyprus again in January 1956 and a further section in June. The remainder arrived in August, joining the operations against the EOKA Terrorists.

In November 1956 part of the Twenty-Third PFA landed in Egypt for the Suez Campaign, the remainder landed by sea. They stayed until the withdrawal, under United Nations supervision, on 22nd December 1956.

The stories of the Airborne Medical Services will continue, with members of the Royal Army Dental Corps playing their part with the Airborne Field Ambulances. We can look back with proud remembrance, of those members of our corps who have worn the Red Beret, the Pegasus Badge, and the Red Cross Brassard.

MY INTRODUCTION TO THE ARMY DENTAL CORPS

[Captain D. H. Ridler, MC]

I joined the AD Corps in the first week of November 1939 and was demobilised in early January 1946. During my six years of service, I was captured three times, recaptured twice, escaped once, dropped twice by parachute into enemy-occupied territory, visited four countries, two islands – Sicily and Malta – was torpedoed, and received a gong! I do not think many in the Dental Corps could have had so varied or interesting a war.

My first posting was to the dental centre in Brecon, the depot of the South Wales Borderers. In the winter of 1939 it was a cold bleak place, and my vivid memory is of the batman bringing my early morning tea, and when I came to drink it, it was frozen solid.

The second posting was to the 195th Field Ambulance, then stationed at Stock, near Billericay in Essex. This was just as Dunkirk was being evacuated and was soon followed by the Battle of Britain. As this raged overhead, the field ambulance, which was part of the Fifteenth Scottish Division, prepared for the German invasion and I was introduced to the practice of dentistry in field conditions.

I do not think the equipment contained in the field panniers had been updated since the 1914-18 war. It was basic and practical, but the collapsible chair was a monstrosity and the foot engine did not encourage much conservative work. Nevertheless, the Deputy Assistant Director of the Dental Service (DADDS) got his monthly treatment statistical return and there were few rockets. I was later to bless the wirecutting capacity of some of the instruments contained in the panniers, when the time came to escape after Arnhem.

The field ambulance gradually moved northwards up through East Anglia, and the Headquarters Company was usually in some Georgian mansion. As the threat of invasion passed, the Fifteenth Scottish Division, which was a Territorial one, was reformed and the field ambulance transferred to the Seventieth Division which had a coastal defence role.

I thought it was time for a change, and when on leave I paid a visit to my old CO, who was a Regular RAMC Officer and was now in the higher echelon of the Army Medical Directorate (AMD) in the War Office. He mentioned that a parachute field ambulance was being formed, and I asked whether there would be a dental officer on its strength, and if so I would like to volunteer.

Sixteenth (Parachute) Field Ambulance – First Parachute Brigade

I was posted to the embryo Sixteenth (P) Field Ambulance and reported at Hardwick Hall near Chesterfield on 4th April 1942. It was not long after the successful raid on the radiolocation station at Bruneval and there was a tremendous spirit in the camp. It was just as well that I was fairly fit on joining. The 195th Field Ambulance had just had a cross-country race at the HQ Company, which was looked down upon by A and P Companys as unfit desk-wallahs, who had run them off the map. I made the effort for HQ Company and was proud to have been the first officer home and to have beaten Peter Candler, the English International Rugby centre three-quarter.

At Hardwick we were hit by an intensive fortnight of PT – runs, forced marches, jumping off scaffolding, and session after session of climbing a platform some eight feet high. We had to sit round a hole which represented the exit hole of a Whitley bomber, jumping through with knees and feet together, and rolling away before the next man landed on your head. At the end of the day there was little conversation in the Mess, groans predominating and bed beckoned early.

The training culminated in descents from a tower. A steel cable, wound round a drum, was attached to the harness of the jumper who then leapt from the platform. As he fell, his weight caused the drum to revolve, its speed being checked by two vanes which created an air-break as they revolved.

At that time, all parachute troops were volunteers and few failed the course.

I had previously met one of the medical officers, Jock McGavin, having played against him in a Hospitals' Cup rugby match. He was a man of granite, and suggested that rather than go by train with the rest of the unit to Ringway, Manchester, it would do us far more good to walk there.

It was a long fifty-four miles, but we set out from Hardwick after lunch on the Saturday, slept in a barn along the way, and strode over tops of the Peak District next morning. I think we did it to impress our new CO, but he was a man of granite too, and I do not think we collected many brownie points.

Parachute training at Ringway was the responsibility of the RAF, and the field ambulance was divided up into small sticks of ten under the instruction of an RAF Sergeant. These instructors were staff recruited from the Physical Training Branch of the RAF and all had completed upwards of forty jumps.

The confidence they inspired was quite unforgettable. The atmosphere at Ringway was in stark contrast to that at Hardwick. The food was superb and we were waited upon by smiling young WAAFs. We were cosseted. The first days of the training there were much as at Hardwick, although some of the apparatus was more sophisticated.

The Whitley bomber was still being used as the dropping vehicle, and our first two jumps from the balloon were through a hole which simulated the exit hole of the Whitley. Balloon jumping is a truly traumatic experience. The instructor and four trainees climb into the basket, which sways gently on takeoff. The drum pays out the cable and it vibrates gently, until at 600ft it stops and there is utter silence. Number One sits with his feet in the hole, and on the command pushes off with his hands to drop 120ft, before his momentum is sufficient to open the parachute. These three seconds are terrifying.

After that, life is heavenly until a voice from below reminds Number One that "You are going backwards – turn around," or "You have somersaulted – get your feet out of the rigging lines."

The Whitley was a dreadful aeroplane. It looked like a flying coffin, and the interior resembled one – dark, cramped and bare. We were encouraged by our instructor that in an emergency it could fly on one engine. "Just as well," he said. "One fell off the other day!"

However, it was a great improvement on the balloon jump, as one's parachute opened almost immediately in the slipstream. I did my seven jumps and an extra one as there was a vacancy in a 'stick'.

This was a mistake, as a breeze got up as I left the aircraft and it took me into a wood on the edge of the dropping zone. Luckily I was able to climb down my leg-straps and fall on the soft ground below.

It was a great moment when we received our 'Wings' and our 'Red Berets'.

The field ambulance assembled at Bulford Camp at the beginning of May. On the first morning we were woken by the sound of concentrated small-arms fire. The German invasion had not begun, but a rabbit had inadvisedly appeared outside the windows of the officers quarters.

This state of readiness was the hallmark of the First Brigade.

I did no dentistry that summer but was sent on courses in anaesthesia in Lincoln and at Park Prewett, where the great Sir Harold Gillies held sway. I dreaded being let loose on the maestro after being told by the delightful Canadian lady anaesthetist who was instructing me that, on withdrawing an endotracheal tube, Sir Harold spotted a piece of tissue on the end.

"Christ! My uvula," said he.

"My sincere apologies," said she.

The role of the parachute field ambulance dental officer had not been fully appraised. In some quarters it was felt that the AD Corps had just got in on the act and as a result he became something of a dogsbody. I was even sent on a motor-maintenance course at Sandbanks, Poole. However, training, the organisation of the two surgical teams, and the packing of all essential supplies into the dropping containers took up most of our time. We were, after all, the pioneer unit of the Airborne Forces medical department.

We did a few drops on Salisbury Plain, and having watched the American Parachute Brigade 'Walking' out of the doors of Dakotas we were highly impressed and envious.

The field ambulance left Bulford in November and embarked in Greenock for the invasion of North Africa. I was detailed to bring out the reinforcements and the RASC detachment.

I was totally unprepared and untrained for the duties which normal adjutants take in their stride. Some examples: Pte Hill, J., had sold his colt automatic in a pub – Court of Enquiry; Cpl Power, J., had taken the CO's car into Salisbury with a few buddies for a night out – Court Martial? Or will you accept my punishment? The last straw was a very rude letter from the stationmaster at Crewe: Pte Deegan,

F., had been caught without a ticket or pass travelling from Chesterfield to Crewe. Would I remit the fare forthwith?

By this time the Brigade Major was an old friend. He had worked in Fleet Street for a national newspaper. "Shred it all and put it in the bin," was his advice. In early March, when the unit was in a most unhealthy position in the Tumera Valley, being shelled by the enemy, which was trying with some success to enlarge his evacuation area around Bizerte, a despatch rider came up the road after having braved the miles from Brigade Headquarters, and handed one message to the colonel. It was from the stationmaster of Crewe!

The rear details held all the unit's criminals and wide boys. I had a miserable weekend wondering whether they would return from a forty-eight hour pass, we being on notice to move. Thankfully they all did. We embarked from Liverpool in the old Cunarder *Scythia,* sailed up to the Clyde where the convoy assembled, and then out into the Atlantic. The course must have taken us almost to America, and the only break in the monotony was when we were summoned to 'action stations'. It was exciting to pass through the Straits of Gibraltar and see the lights of Spain and Tangiers. Algiers looked beautiful in the early morning sunshine and the *Scythia* anchored in the outer harbour and waited its turn to disembark.

Night fell, and the air raid siren sounded, followed closely by the drone of bombers. There was a Greek cargo vessel astern of us which let off salvo after salvo mostly through our rigging, and then a torpedo struck the *Scythia*, shaking her like one shakes a sauce bottle. The old ship settled down until the bow was just under and the stern high out of the water. My station was dead aft. The scene was enlivened by a destroyer coming close alongside and a very cultured voice saying over the tannoy, *"Scythia, Scythia,* where are you hit?"

"Up the bleeding sharp end – where do you think?" was the shout from the assembled troops. The only casualty was General Eisenhower's staff car.

The winter up in the Tunisian hills was for the most part cold and miserable. After the capture of the port of Bone and the airfield at Souk el Khemis, and a disastrous drop by the Second Battalion, there were no other parachute operations, and the brigade spent the time yo-yoing between the front and Algiers, plugging gaps in the line when the enemy made a thrust.

This journey took almost a week by train and we did it three times by rail and once by sea. This was in a Hunt Class destroyer from

Algiers to Bone, where I was unpleasantly surprised to find the DADDS waiting for me on the quay demanding a return of treatment rendered. The panniers had been opened on occasion and a few teeth extracted. What more could he have expected?

The surgical teams had also been in action when the Americans had to give ground at Depienne. We set up in a large Arab barn and used the absent owner's harem as a Mess. It was a small harem and I slept in a hole burrowed out of a haystack. My neighbour was a gunner acting as an ADP, with his Auster plane hidden between two other stacks. The German Messerschmidts were always over, but although he was often chased he was quite confident that as long as he looked in his mirror and picked them up before they got too close, he could turn far more quickly and fly much lower than they could.

This was my first experience of giving anaesthetics in the field, and the conditions could not have been rougher. We had to rely almost exclusively on Pentothal and ether. Cedric Longland (Shorty) was very patient with his anaesthetist. I was the only one he had!

Between breaks in the action there was the opportunity to explore the country. The farm was at the head of a wide valley and teemed with water fowl, goldfinches and storks. I managed to shoot a teal with an American carbine that one of the GIs had left behind, and my batman cooked it. I also collected a goose and three ducks, one a drake. These I kept in a fifty gallon petrol drum and they became camp followers.

At the beginning of March, the brigade moved to the northern sector of the Tunisian front where the enemy was having his only success in widening his escape route from Bizerte. The surgical teams were kept busy in several locations, including the little port of Tabarka and in the Tamera valley. Here the theatre was in a deserted farm at the head of a marshy valley infested with frogs. They were courting and the noise was deafening.

Conditions were basic and we slept in a rat-infested loft, being wakened by the vermin running along the rafters and sometimes trying to get at the emergency rations in our haversacks, which we used as pillows. Here I extracted a tooth for a legionnaire, who was so grateful that he came back later with a large pig which we roasted, and invited the colonel in for the feast.

Compo rations were beginning to pall by this time. On learning that these pigs were running loose in the valley, I was detailed to round up a few more so that the colonel might impress the brigadier.

This was a disaster, as the truck carrying the three porkers was shot up by a Messerschmidt. The pigs jumped out and ran into a minefield. Two were blown up and the third vanished, never to be seen again.

A few days later, the enemy made a flanking attack and we had to evacuate in a hurry, after operating on several casualties. Sadly there was no room for my farmyard of three ducks and a goose – the three-tonner had room only for the surgical team and the patients. When the enemy was thrown back days later, I searched for my stock but without success. Both the ducks and the goose had been laying and made a good prize.

After the end of the North African Campaign, the field ambulance left Algiers, and on 12th May it made camp just outside the perimeter of an airstrip at Matmore, near Mascara in Western Algeria. (There was a signpost there pointing to Timbuktu!) We were in pup-tents, one to one officer, and one to two ORs, and the standard of comfort was zero. The country was baked dry, being on the edge of the Sahara, and a layer of thick dust covered the airstrip.

A dust storm was generated each time a plane took off and little dust-devil mini whirlwinds swept across the plain. My dental centre was in a small tent and I had to post Cpl Scott (Scotty) as a lookout to warn the patients to shut their mouths tight when one of these approached.

On one occasion the whole tent was lifted bodily and was set down fifty yards away. End of session!

We trained intensively for six weeks, but without any hint of the objective. Both Sardinia and Sicily and even Greece cropped up in the disinformation circulated. One day, to relieve the boredom, I begged a flight in a glider to appreciate how the air-landing brigade of our division went into action.

These WACO gliders were delivered in cartons and assembled on the site with hammers and screwdrivers, mostly of the 'Birmingham' kind! The pilot was an American, and although we had witnessed hundreds of take-offs, they were quite dramatic from the point of view of the occupants of the glider. As the Dakota revved up its engines, it disappeared in a cloud of dust. The towrope tightened, and almost as soon as the plane started taxiing, the glider became airborne with the towrope sagging down into the fog.

The Dakota eventually appeared, staggering up through the brown blanket, and finally cast us off at five thousand feet. The pilot seemed to be testing this glider to destruction; stalling, banking and diving. It was a relief to land and I was grateful for at least having some control of arrival on terra firma, being a paratroop.

The training culminated in *Exercise Cactus,* aptly named, as landing in these prickly pears was a painful experience. It was our first drop from Dakotas and we all agreed that this was a Pullman compared with the old Whitley. I made a hard landing on a hard and stony plain and did not appreciate the long march from the dropping zone.

However, spirits were soon raised when we were joined while resting in a ditch by Regimental Sergeant Major J. C. Lord of the Third Battalion. JC (Jesus Christ to the ORs) was reputed to have the loudest voice in the British Army and I remember sitting on Bulford Hill and watching him drilling the 'punishment squad' half a mile from the parade ground and hearing every command!

Two very scruffy old Arabs came shuffling along the road just as dawn was breaking, and JC jumped to his feet and bawled, "Pick 'em up – left – right – left – right." The effect was dramatic. The two old Arabs straightened up and marched just like guardsmen!

On the 30th June, the Sixteen (P) Field Ambulance flew in Dakotas to an airstrip near Sousse in Tunisia. It was an interesting flight, skirting the Sahara, but we were hardly prepared for the heat which hit us as we climbed out of the plane. It was like a solid wall. We settled into an olive grove and suffered the various winds which blow from the desert and which go by various names: the Sirocco, the Khamsin, the Harmattan. They were all bloody hot! However, nearby were the beaches where we could relax and get horribly burnt!

The object of our training was soon revealed, and sand-tables and maps appeared which we had to memorise. The task allotted to the First Parachute Brigade was to capture the long iron lattice-work bridge over the River Simeto, just to the South of Catania, with its vital airfields. It was General Montgomery's fond hope to storm up the coastal plain to Messina over this Primasole Bridge rather than through the mountains to the west of Etna. The Field Ambulance was to set up the Medical Dressing Station in a farm just south of this bridge.

The invasion of Sicily began on the night of 9/10th July with the glider-borne units of the Air-Landing Brigade. It was nearly a complete fiasco, as most of the tug-planes were Dakotas piloted by the Americans, who had never experienced any shooting in anger. At the first bursts they took immediate evading action, many casting off their gliders over the sea. However, the surprise and the skeleton of the brigade was enough to capture the objectives.

The First Brigade was scheduled to drop on D+2, the night of 11/12th July. We were all emplaned when the order came to stand down as the weather was unsuitable. All that adrenalin wasted! The next afternoon we were assured that the operation was on and we again set off for the airstrip. We emplaned and taxied to the end of the runway, and with a loud bang the tyre of the tail wheel exploded. Another setback? No! The Yanks had a special jack for just this occasion. A new wheel was fitted all within twenty minutes and we were on our way, a tail-end Charlie if ever there was one.

We now had to rely on the navigator, and only afterwards did it transpire that there was only one in the formation, in the lead aircraft. The course was laid to the east end of Malta where a cone of searchlights pointed towards the heavens. Afterwards it was a question of flying on a bearing for so many minutes to the mouth of the Simeto, turning sharp to port, and dropping almost immediately.

The surgeon, Captain Lippman-Kessell, RAMC, was in command of the plane-load of twenty, his surgical team. He became uneasy as the plane droned on and he looked out of the port window and saw Mount Etna broad on the port beam. He tapped the so-called navigator on the shoulder, who then tapped the pilot on his and shouted, "Jeez! We've gone too far! Turn the ship around, Captain!" This he did, and we flew over the straits of Messina and out to sea in a huge circle, coming in again over the coast, very, very low. The pilot had warned us at the briefing that he would do this and we had to be prepared to hold on tightly as he shot up to dropping height.

We picked out a gun crew on the ground, tracer came up and there was a smell of burning. The pilot made the steepest climb of his life, and we who were standing all went down like a line of lead soldiers. By the time we had struggled to our feet, on came the green light, and as Number One of the stick I jumped. I was glad to get out after the tension which had been building up since leaving Malta.

It was a beautiful cool night: moonless, but with enough light from the fires burning on the ground to see that it was flat. For once I made a good landing on soft earth, and by the light of a burning haystack I walked down the line and gathered up the men and the containers. We were four short – Numbers Seventeen, Eighteen,

Nineteen and Twenty – and Twenty was Lippy. Our CO, Number Sixteen, said that when the green light came on, the man behind him had collapsed and perhaps impeded the others. He might have been hit by ground fire.

With great good fortune, the RSM was in the stick. RSM Brock was a quiet, solid and utterly reliable man who was very popular in the unit. We also has an RASC Corporal, another rock of a man but with a stutter which went well with the Sten gun he carried. I hid the men and all the equipment in a haystack and took the RSM off to reconnoitre and try to pick some feature we might recognise from the sand-table.

Mount Etna with its snow-cap stood out to the north of us, so that was a plus. We thought that there was an embankment to the west, and if so it must be a railway. If the guess was correct, we were only a few miles off the dropping zone. We went back to the men and they were all fast asleep. I never ceased to marvel at their capacity for switching off when under stress.

We reckoned that the course to the bridge was to the east and set off with the trolleys, carrying the equipment. It was hard and frustrating progress, as deep ditches crossed the plain every few hundred yards. There would also be ghostly figures emerging with guns at the ready. Challenging us with the password, "Desert Rats", which had to be answered, "Kill Italians".

Fortunately, these were all lost souls of the First Brigade who had been dropped away from their zones. We soon collected about ten of these souls, who seemed to have greater faith in our bump of locality than they had in theirs. When we at last came to the embankment of the Gornalunga Canal, they found that their faith had been justified, and I delivered them to Brigade HQ with some relief.

We were now close to the southern end of the Primasole Bridge and all we had to do was to go up the road, take the first on the left and then another three hundred yards down to the farm on the left. As we walked up the road, a ghostly figure emerged from a ditch and warned us that an Italian tank was moving up and down the road. Before we had gone more than a few yards, there was an extraordinary grinding noise in the distance and this apparition, spouting sparks, appeared behind us.

We hurriedly took to the ditch and waved it past. It was still dark, but the first streaks of dawn were appearing. We then turned left and met some friends of the First Battalion who had captured a farm on

58

the right-hand side of the road. I enquired whether anybody had been
down the road to the farm on the left some two hundred yards away.
Nobody had, so we proceeded.

At the farm entrance, I halted the men and went on with Corporal
Power of the stutter and Sten gun. A figure emerged and challenged
us in Italian, but after a few shots in his direction, which fortunately
did not hit him, he threw down his rifle. There were then stirrings in
the large barn and I told Power to fire a long blast through the door.
Our sentry told his mates that their war was over and the upstairs
windows flew open and a shower of rifles descended on us. Cpl
Power lined up the guard, about twenty strong, and the RSM and I
inspected the farm.

It had seven rooms and a small kitchen and was indescribably
dirty. The RSM set our prisoners to work with brooms and
scrubbers, while I went back to the First Battalion to try and get some
picture of the situation. It was getting light and some of the braver
Italians were creeping up and taking pot-shots, luckily with little
effect. I was soon joined by Cedric Longland, our senior surgeon,
who had experienced the same difficulties with the ditches and
trolleys. I was very glad to see him and his team and took him down
to the farm, which was now less of an Augean stable.

He and the RSM then went about organising the building into the
MDS. We now had a reception centre, a pre-operative room,
operating theatre, two post-operative rooms, and three wards. While
I was busy with the unpacking, the padre of the First Brigade came to
me and said, "There's a large party of Italians coming up the road,
and I don't know if they are friendly." I gave him my Colt
automatic, and Padre Watkins stood at the farm entrance and waved
them in. We soon had the whole farmyard full and I felt they would
burst into an operatic chorus at any minute.

We were greatly heartened when Colonel Wheatley, our CO,
came riding in on a bicycle. Ross Wheatley was greatly loved and
later became a Major-General and Chief Surgeon to the Army. Now
we were able to man the two surgical teams and we were soon in
business with casualties, British, German and Italian. The day
became hotter and hotter.

After one case I realised that my anaesthetist's stool was in fact a
small barrel. It did not take long to find that it was full of quite
passable Chianti – the rations of the dispossessed Italian guard.
Drinking wine out of mess tins might scandalise any self-respecting

sommelier, but it kept us happy and working that long day as the battle raged outside.

There was much small-arms fire, but only two shells landed near the farm without doing any damage. My dental corporal, Scott (Scotty), put in some very gallant and hazardous work, collecting casualties from crashed gliders and from the Regimental Aid Posts. He wondered why there were so many bees about which he couldn't see. He soon realised that a sniper had him in his sights, and Scotty hurriedly took cover. He showed great initiative, capturing a horse and cart to provide transport for his casualties.

Late in the afternoon, the fortunes of war turned against us when the Germans brought up eighty-eight millimetre guns and began to blast the pill boxes at the end of the bridge. When dusk fell, the MDS was in no man's land, and after a fairly quiet night an Italian major stalked in and announced that we were all captured and would be evacuated. As none of our team had more than a few Italian swear words between us, the CO, knowing that I had a smattering of French and German, told me to chat him up while the rest of the MDS went on working.

The major was impressed to find that we had been operating on Italians and German troops as well as our own, and he soon realised the impossibility of moving them without a convoy of ambulances, which of course he did not have. I told him that General Montgomery was just up the road, and as if in answer to a prayer a heavy gun opened up and an armour-piercing shell hit the bridge with a noise like a gigantic jew's harp.

The Major really did think it was Monty, took the hint and left. We found out later that our Royal Engineers had removed all the demolition charges as soon as the bridge was taken, and as a last resort the Germans were trying to destroy it by gunfire. They even strung up a large bomb to the parapet but could not explode it. We were interested onlookers to all these goings-on and were soon recaptured by our own First and Second Battalions, and later the forward troops of the Fiftieth (Northumbrian) Division.

The casualties continued to arrive, including our own Brigadier Lathbury. It was with some trepidation that I gave him pentothal while Shorty Longland removed fragments of a mortar shell. The MDS closed soon after 1700 hours and we were evacuated some miles behind the fighting. The MDS had treated a hundred and nine casualties, there were thirty-five operations completed and only two

60

post-operative deaths. During the operation we had captured a beautiful Italian ambulance and a large brand-new Lancia lorry.

I persuaded the CO to let me stay and clear much of the equipment, which was still lying on the dropping zones. With a sergeant, a driver and another, we loaded over a hundred parachutes, Vickers guns, Stens, blood and plasma, and anything else which came to hand. We had to be pulled out of a ditch one night by an armoured car and then were persecuted by the most virulent mosquitoes. That night, a company of a Yorkshire Regiment came past us and enquired as to what exactly we were doing. The captain was Hedley Verity, the left-arm England slow-bowler and one of my heroes. He was killed that night leading his company.

We took all our salvage back to Syracuse and were stopped by General Montgomery en route. I saluted as smartly as I knew how and received a parcel of cigarettes and some words of encouragement from the great man. I do not smoke, but I knew that Victory V cigarettes were of dubious Indian origin, and was not surprised that my rear-party received them with less than enthusiasm.

In Syracuse I saw a notice for a Medical Inspection Room and went inside to find a very harassed and short-tempered MO. I asked him whether he would like a Roll Royce of an ambulance, as I was giving one away. I got a fairly rude answer, but he brightened up when he saw the beauty.

Soon after we had dropped on the night of 12/13th and while we were trying to locate our position, the RSM and I were intrigued by persistent squeaking noises coming from the west, where we thought the railway should have been. When clearing the dropping zone, we ventured to the railway and found under a bridge a load of German parachute equipment together with some of their trolleys. These were the squeakers. The German Brigade had dropped on the same zone as we had but some little time before. We had had a narrow escape.

AWARD OF THE MILITARY CROSS – CITATION

Captain D. H. Ridler, MC, AD Corps (Sicily)
The official citation states:
"On the night of July 13th, 1943, Captain Ridler was dropped by parachute near the Ponte Primasole. He led his *stick* with heavy equipment on a trolley over four miles of difficult country. Captain

Ridler entered the farm selected as a dressing station with one combatant soldier, who took prisoner twenty Italian soldiers who were occupying it. He set his men and the prisoners to prepare the dressing station and himself went off to contact other units.

For two days he worked in the dressing station under fire, giving anaesthetics for two surgeons. It was by his initiative and gallantry that the dressing station was set up, and by his devotion to duty that operations were able to be performed even when the dressing station was overrun by the enemy."

A DENTIST AT WAR
1939-1945
[William Herbert Edmonds, LDS U.
Birmingham 1942]

In late August 1939, when I was at the Birmingham Medical School, having just completed Anatomy and Physiology, it was decided that a First Aid Station would be set up in the basement. Students and staff would man the same. All normal studies ceased. We began by sandbagging the basement windows. Those of you who know the school will realise that this was a somewhat arduous task. Some senior staff had been in the First World War and to begin with; these people instructed on the First Aid Manual of the RAMC of that time – triangular bandages, and so on.

The basement had been cleared of all objects except for the loos and urinals and substituted by rows of stretchers. By 1st September we were in full-time occupation, sleeping on stretchers at night, and receiving food sent in from the university – we were probably some fifty altogether.

It turned out that of these personnel there were only two of us who had even the basic skills of cooking – B. O. M. Norris (in the year ahead of me) and myself. Thus it was, that on the morning of 3rd September, he and I were cooking sixteen pounds of beef in the gas cooker of the Pathology Laboratory (having first removed the remaining trays which had been used for incubation and washing it out).

At eleven o'clock we heard Neville Chamberlain's speech to the nation. We had clubbed together to buy a pint bottle of brown ale and what with the heat of the small room and the news, we thought it was an appropriate time to remove the cap and wish each other good luck.

Albert Russell, the University Tailors, were commissioned to supply First Aiders with badges, like miniature blazer badges, which we pinned on our lapels. It was a tense time which turned out to be the 'Phoney War', and after a month or so we resumed our studies.

My year was split up into two sections – one half went at night to be fire watches at the old dental hospital in Great Charles Street, and the other half, of which I was one, did three nights a week in what had been the cycle sheds at the Edgbaston University buildings, as First Aiders. This was built very substantially of stone and concrete, and we shared it with the Auxiliary Fire Service. The Chief Fireman was the Head Porter of the Union (Students). His two under-porters were his second in command and leading fireman respectively, with a few more from the remainder of them who looked after the buildings.

We got into a very happy routine – a telephone was put in so that we could receive an amber, green or red warning of enemy planes. It wasn't easy to do any study on these nights on duty, because there was the noise of cards being played – brag, dominoes, and pontoon. The pub – The Gun Barrels – was also nearby, so, as was so often at this time of war, we could nip down for a pint because we were in telephone contact if a warning came through.

The months went by and then an amber warning came through – then, ten minutes later, the red. We soon heard the "brrm brrm" of the twin-engined bombers of these days. It was quite a concentrated raid on Birmingham. Two planes came over Edgbaston buildings and dropped sticks of fire bombs. We all turned out from the cycle sheds, kicked the sticks, put clods of earth from the rose beds on them – all quite contrary to our instructions. I was by this time quite near the Barber Institute when a few more planes came over and dropped high explosive bombs. One was quite near but I was fortunate – the blast only partially debagged me!

Students went on, air raids went on, but fortunately we never had to treat a patient needing First Aid.

At this time I was studying Dental Mechanics, Dental Anatomy and Dental Pathology. When exam time came, I had a great bit of good luck with my oral in Dental Anatomy. My godmother, mother's sister, was matron of a nursing home in Northampton and she was a friend of the chief constable. A child's skull had been dug up during some building operation – not enough to require an inquest – and this had come to me through the post! I had drilled away the lower jaw to expose the permanent teeth growing underneath the baby teeth and this had been put in the Medical School's museum.

When I went into the examination room, the external examiner picked up this very specimen from the variety of teeth from the whole human and animal kingdom which were laid out before him and handed it to me to discuss! I am sure the internal examiner gave me a wink. I could have told him where it was dug up. I just managed to pass.

So the clinical year passed – two years in all. This was much more rewarding now we were doing proper dentistry. Our equipment was very primitive compared with modern times. Students had a foot treadle drill and an instrument cabinet all supplied at our parents' expense. There were three electrically-driven drills, two in the demonstration rooms and one in the surgical room. We envied these quite a lot! There was only one bursary a year in those days to help with students' expenses, but there was a great help from the honorary dental surgeons who gave their time free to teach us not only the practical side of dentistry, but to listen to a patient, be it about their teeth or family worries. We were very lucky!

So I managed to qualify towards the end of 1942 and became a Registered LDS on December 7th of that year.

While awaiting my call-up papers I did various locum jobs. The papers came with a uniform allowance and I became very smart with my uniform swagger stick, brown gloves and two pips on my shoulder! I went to the Dental School to bid my farewells and happened to bump into the Dean, Colonel Howkings. When I told him I had been posted to Aldershot, he revealed that he had taken his Major's certificate there. He said that it was very convenient for popping up to London – you could have a night out, return on the early train, and be back on parade early next morning. "Known as the Fornicating Special, my boy."

So I proceeded to the Mecca of the military – Aldershot. Three of our year had been posted there, and thanks to Philip Hughes we all met at his father's cottage near Abingdon – Philip, Stan Bollington, and myself. They couldn't have been nicer – we all tried on our uniforms. I had not had delivery of my Sam Browne – only a cloth belt. On the Monday morning we reported to Aldershot and I joined a six-officer dental centre in Knollys Road.

So there I was – a lieutenant with two pips on my shoulder – and after two weeks I felt a proper twerp, still not knowing how to return a salute in the proper manner. I asked the CO – was there not an instruction centre to learn such things? He replied that I had to wait six weeks until we had such a course. However, he kindly arranged for me to be relieved of dental duties one morning a week for me to have instruction in drill and saluting! It made a change from teeth and I felt a much more competent officer of His Majesty's Forces.

In due course I was posted to the fourteen day course, and because of my previous experience of drill I was made Right Marker when we went on parade. I learned map reading and the theory of wiring jaws. Then the Passing Out Parade – I was Right Marker and had I obeyed the Drill Lieutenant, everything would have gone adrift. However, I did not mind ending up Left Man in the rear rank. I used my common sense and the CO congratulated us all on being the best parade officers he had ever seen. First lesson in the army: use your own initiative within the orders you are given!

I was then posted to East Kent District – Maidstone – the Thirteenth I.T.C. Having reported, I then had to find lodgings. The ones I found were in Sandling, not far from The Running Horse Inn – a fortunate choice. This was, of course, a restricted zone for people going in and out. I can remember the husband's name (Rex) but not his wife's, but they were very good to me. You must appreciate the times we lived in – constant air attacks and rationing – but the spirit of everyone was, "we will beat those bloody Huns".

The Dental Centre was a six-chair one, commanded by a TA, Major Gerry – from Barnstaple – a nicer man you could never meet. Every intake to the training centre had a six week basic instruction, and we were supposed to make their teeth fit during that time. This was very hard work, non-stop every day, both mentally and physically tiring. I remember one day we had an inspection from the ADDS (Assistant Director of the Army Dental Service) – a tall bloke who, when he entered the surgery, put a hand on the top of the door to see if there was any dust on it, while carrying on a conversation with the dentist working in the surgery. One newly-joined one, working in his battledress trousers and white operating gown, came smartly to a salute instead of standing to attention, one of his canvas gaiters having fallen on the floor. Of course, you never salute the King with your hat off and I wonder where this officer was posted to – the Inspecting Officer was not best pleased! (He turned up in a Worcester practice after the war.)

One intake, all in their civvies and with fibre attaché cases, came through the gates manned by guards in their guard house – one man had painted on his case 'Slasher Green'. He only stayed on the camp forty-eight hours before breaking out – never to be seen again while I was there.

Gerry, the CO, was billeted with the local Ministry vet and his wife (John and Vera Stewart). Like all Scots they were very hospitable and invited me to join them at home whenever I had any free time. There was another family – I think their name was Brooke Ellis – on the other side of Maidstone, who owned a paper mill mainly producing the thin paper for those lovely old five pound notes. Their house was called Turkey Court, and one day a notice was pinned up on the notice board inviting any officer who would like to join them for Sunday tea to phone them. I took advantage of this kind offer, borrowed an army bicycle, and proceeded to the other side of town. They were the nicest people, and not only did I stay to tea but had supper as well – my companion was a French officer.

I always remember these meals – they had their own hens and the omelette we had for the four of us had twelve eggs in it. When you think of the hard times and rationing in 1943, this was the most luxurious meal I had had since leaving home.

I had been keen on fishing since I was a young boy, and when I was told that three ponds that fed the water mill to make their machine work were stocked with fish, I was more than interested. It thus turned out that I was invited to catch some pike in the top pond the following Sunday. I could hardly concentrate on the next week's extractions and fillings. Come the next Sunday, I got on my bike, and found the punt ready for me. The gardener had caught some roach for me and they were in a live bait can with the rod, line, float and hooks all at the ready! One did not think in those days of the cruelty of this kind of fishing. You put two hooks through the top of the fish's back, cast it out, and waited for the float to dip. You can describe a pike as a freshwater shark. It will always take a fish horizontally – all its teeth are curved backwards so you have to be patient while it turns the fish longways on, in order to swallow it, and you have to count to twenty before you drive home the hooks.

Enough to say that I cycled home, not only full of another omelette but with two pike on the carrier. Having told the Stewarts of my expedition, they said that if I was successful I should call in and Vera would cook them for the next night. This became a regular date on Mondays. After the fish supper, which was a great addition to our mundane diet, we played cards or poker dice.

You must remember that we lived from day to day. German bombers came over night after night, and indeed one night one was shot down and crashed in a nearby field. We all drank too much beer and I remember one evening after supper the two next door neighbours came in and we played strip poker. I can't remember who suggested this, but I had been forewarned and I put on a pair of bathing trunks. It was abandoned (not the bathing trunks) at two a.m. all square.

It had been an early spring and I even remember sitting in a deck chair on a couple of occasions. Then a posting order came through that I was to go to a dental centre in Edinburgh. I packed up, collected a travel warrant, left Maidstone for London – King's Cross – for the night train north. Officers always had a first-class warrant but on this occasion, owing to the shortage of rolling stock, I had to stand in the corridor the whole way.

This was the first time I went to sleep standing on my feet – an asset I learned early on, and had to use on future occasions. I was not exactly at my best when we drew into Waverley Station at 7.30 a.m. I ascended the famous (or should I say infamous) Waverley steps with my raincoat on my arm, carrying my suitcase, and met a blistering east wind – the contrast from Kent was great.

I enquired where Colinton was, took the tram along Princes Street, at the end of which was another tram which would take me there and by midday I had reported for duty at my new dental centre, only to be informed that there was no accommodation in the nearby Officers' Mess. However, my new CO phoned the Billeting Officer and at 6 p.m. I ended up at the Church of Scotland hostel in the Haymarket District. I was informed that I could stay for one week while looking for digs.

Four weeks later and still there, I was offered and gratefully took an attic room in the Marchment area. Just a skylight from which to see the daylight, and every breakfast was porridge and herrings (I've not eaten a herring since but still enjoy porridge on a cold winter morning). The cost for this privilege was 35/- a week which was quite high in those days for B and B.

While living at the hostel and after a long day's dentistry, I retired to the bar of the Grosvenor Hotel which was nearby. It had been commandeered for Government purposes, but the ground floor bar and restaurant were still free for normal service. This bar was a long L-shaped one and it was a six o'clock meeting place for officers of East Scotland Headquarters where we used to enjoy a couple of pints before finding something to eat. Dorothy was the barmaid – not the most Scottish of names – but a most cheerful girl until the first Americans came to help in our war!

Immediately a notice went up to say that we only have liqueur whisky at so much a measure – an increase of a hundred percent. Poor allies! They did not mind as they always had rolls of pound notes in rubber bands in their pockets and proceeded to order a dozen large ones.

Bateman would have made a good sketch of our faces. Memory lets me down but I think a full lieutenant got £1/10/- a week then. At our next six o'clock meeting I noticed that the assistant barmaid was putting a bottle of whisky on the sink and scrubbing off the label, then putting it behind the liqueur whisky bottles. It so happened that it was my turn to buy the next round. Dorothy was serving me this time and I jokingly said, "I'm going to have to black on you. I saw what happened, and how dare you treat our allies like that!"

I saw her face change colour from a ruddy hue to ashen white and wondered if I might be called to attend to a fainting barmaid. She recovered her composure, went to the pumps and drew our beers. I put 2/- on the counter and received 2/6d change! This established custom went on for several weeks. Did she really think I was going to put the black on her? Typically, my state of bliss at having free beer every night after a hard day's work helped me face those awful herrings with all their bones very morning, was about to change.

A posting order came through – I was going to the Boom Defence HQ in the Orkneys. Once again, I packed my bag and took the train north. This was a very civilised journey, compared with the one from Kent – a first-class compartment and no changes all the way to N.E. Scotland. The scenery was magnificent and it was a wonderful day off from churning out all those target fillings.

The train arrived at Thurso when dawn was breaking over the harbour. The usual formalities of movement orders were checked, and I embarked. I think I am right in saying that those supply ships were about four hundred tons. A grey misty morning with an increasing wind, the engines revved, lines were cast off and we left the bay. I, together with members of all three services, was enjoying a cup of coffee when all hell was let loose.

The captain must have known something, because guard rails had been put around the tables to stop the crockery rolling off the tables. Soon, not only were the cups and saucers on the floor, but we were too! I have never known such a terrifying sea journey. I was the only semi-medical aboard. Ths ship did everything, but thankfully it did not sink! Instead of being a four hour trip it took nearly twelve hours before we reached the calmer waters of Scapa Flow and tied up at Stromness.

Everyone was being sick all over the place – even the naval officers. I had to deal with three broken arms, two broken legs, and numerous other injuries. It took forty-eight hours to repair the ship before it could return to Thurso.

So there I was, completely shattered, reporting to the Movement Officer, who said that he had got a fifteen cwt truck taking stores to the Boom Defence – with my suitcase I sat in a privileged place by the driver. The rain was lashing down, but the wind was beginning to abate. The base was halfway between Stromness and Kirkwall and I was even expected! My duties were to look after the naval personnel and the ack-ack batteries defending them. I was shown to my room and a naval steward came to introduce himself. He said, "I hear you have had a bit of a rough passage. I expect you would like a hot bath. I will go and draw one for you." What bliss! I nearly went to sleep in it.

The next morning I reported to the naval commander – a cheery RN who warmly welcomed even a Brown Job, and showed me into a superb one-chair surgery and introduced me to my male naval assistant. It was a great joy – no pressure and doing the job I was trained for. For the next week I caught up with the backlog of work left by my predecessor.

I then asked for transport to take me to visit the ack-ack batteries I was to look after and arranged times for them to come and have their teeth inspected and treated. They were very ready to have any diversion – even a dental one! They had to be at full alertness day and night.

In the third week, an ENSA party came to entertain them and I was invited to this show. Again, transport was laid on and my eventual memory of this event is somewhat hazy. Both artists (?) and myself were invited back to the Gunner's Mess where the beer flowed. I vaguely remember pouring some of mine into the shoe of one of the female artistes who had done a skit on *Cinderella*. I asked for her shoe, poured beer into it, and we both drank to the end of the war!

I had been treating some of the crew of the three MTBs who were on standby with their depth charges in case of another submarine attack. They invited me for Sunday drinks. They were moored alongside each other with gangplanks from the quay to the first and connecting the others. Their plan of attack was to give you a very large gin (duty free, of course, at 2d a time), and then you moved slightly more warily to the second and third boat. By twelve o'clock we were swaying somewhat and had to return to the quay across the aforesaid gangplanks. I followed the naval officer's position in front of me – namely crawling along on all fours, in order to avoid a trip into the waters below, and learned why they are called the Senior Service – showing such initiative under difficult conditions!

Transported back to our own Mess we then had a vast Sunday lunch. Food was available to keep the Navy going, and I can still picture the commander remonstrating with the steward for not bringing a steel to sharpen the carving knife before he tackled the roast beef. Life was good. Like most people, we smoked cigarettes and my steward used to bring me packets from an opposite number on one of the ships lying in the Scapa – duty free. It was, of course, too good to last – after only four and a half weeks I was ordered back to Aldershot.

We left Stromness at dusk – a beautiful night with an almost full moon – no wind, and the anger of the Pentland Firth had gone to sleep. I had just settled into my cabin when there was a tap on the door. I was informed that I was the Senior Army Officer on board. I was in charge of all troops and was invited to inspect and count them from the boarding list – a little different from looking in peoples' mouths.

It couldn't have been more of a contrast, this journey – the sea was like a millpond. There was a brief interlude of luxury, travelling first-class as an officer was entitled to, and when I eventually reported back to where this story began, I was told that I was being posted abroad. This was all top secret. I was given seven days' leave and went home to my loving parents in Birmingham who, of course, I could not tell that I might not see them for a little while!

As you can imagine, all the goodies that had been put away for me were revealed and it was a lovely relaxing week.

Back to Aldershot to be fitted out with tropical kit, including, as an officer, a canvas bag with collapsible frame, a folding chair with canvas seat and backrest, some nearly-fitting khaki shorts, tunics and long stockings. This lasted forty-eight hours and then we were entrained at night and in secrecy, and puffed away. Next morning we got off the train on a quayside and were directed to the gangplank of a ship moored alongside.

On board we were informed that we were at Liverpool, aboard a troopship and shown into quarters – officers in two-tiered bunks and other ranks below had hammocks. It was a bit of a relief to know where we were, such was the secrecy and blackout conditions of the time. Some time in the night I was woken by the throb of the engines. I tossed and turned in my bunk, and when I woke up it was a lovely October day and a comparatively smooth sea. On the right-hand side there was land in the distance (I had not learned what port and starboard meant).

The coastline disappeared but reappeared some hours later, and we were sailing up a wide estuary where we anchored. It turned out to be Gourock, near Glasgow, although we were not told so at the time. A lot of other ships came and moored around. An announcement came over the tannoy that at various collecting points we could pick up free OHMS postcards that would be posted to our relatives. These were printed buff cards with stereotyped messages – 'I love you', 'See you soon', 'Won't see you soon', etc. You ticked your message, then were able to put your Christian name, saying (as I did) "love from Bill" to my parents.

Again, during the night, the engines began to throb and we set off to our still unknown destination. We were out at sea with many other vessels – ours was a troop carrier and naval vessels were going around at top speed. We had three practices of going to boat stations, putting on lifebelts and instructions how we would abandon ship – a really uplifting start to our unknown destination. So to our bunks to get what sleep we could.

On deck the next morning it was again a nice day and an impressive sight with so many ships. After I had walked the deck to get some exercise, it was my turn for breakfast – pilchards in tomato sauce instead of those Edinburgh herrings. We had a briefing on what our duties would be on the voyage. This was interrupted by the tannoy for boat stations – you can imagine the tension.

We had an Oerlikon gun at the back of the ship and this started up with its noisy fire, and destroyers were going full out all around us. There was a submarine about in the Irish Sea! I shall never know why the Oerlikon was being fired but perhaps it was just practice in case it was a coordinated attack with Junkers. After a couple of hours we returned to our briefing, having stowed away our life jackets.

This ship was an old troopship and on her we sailed on and on. After a somewhat frightening beginning it was a very relaxing time – in those days you lived from day to day. My duties were minimal. There was no dental surgery aboard, but there was plenty of reading matter. The fresh sea air and the exercise around the deck was stimulating, as were the sea water baths – even with sea water soap you could not get a lather.

The days went by with no more red alerts. We noticed one day that there were very few ships around, and then one morning we saw a tip of land with a high peak on the skyline which I immediately recognised as Gibraltar. An hour or two later we sailed into the harbour. Here we took on water and were provisioned. Several new officers came aboard and after a few hours we were making our way across the Mediterranean. This was the first convoy to do so, rather than making its way all around South Africa. Eventually we arrived at Suez.

While awaiting permission to sail through the canal, the ship was surrounded by bum boats offering their wares. A few people succumbed to their sales talk – goods were then hauled up on the ropes they threw to the ship but they were very disappointed with their purchases. Nothing came up to the value of the money they had thrown down. But it was a bit of light relief after the tension of the previous few weeks.

We were warm in our stiff khaki shorts, tunics, long stockings and highly polished brown shoes (black boots for ORs) and as we sailed down the canal we were issued with pith helmets and spine pads to keep us fit in the heat (an issue which went back to the First World War). It was a fascinating time, added to the fact that no one was going to attack us – Port Said, Cairo, Port Toufik. For a young man who had only travelled as far as Wales from his Birmingham home and with all the historical implications of what I saw with my own eyes to be so fascinating – death and destruction were forgotten by all of us.

We sailed on and were informed that we were going to India – the first convoy to go by this route since the submarine menace had been overcome. We had lessons in Urdu – mainly on how to give orders to the natives – a leftover from the British Raj. The route went on – walks around the deck before breakfast, so-called 'stimulating' mandatory lectures by anyone who could try and do same, physical jerks for ORs so that they might get some sleep in their hammocks. We had only brief bulletins of what was happening in the rest of the world. We had agreed with our American allies when they joined the war that troopships of both countries would be 'dry', so we only had lemonade, which was useful for quenching thirst as it got hotter and hotter.

We saw our first flying fish, which broke the monotony and continued to do so. Most people had read and reread all the paperbacks and the food was continuing in its basic way – sufficient to keep you going, but becoming boring. It was suddenly announced that in twenty-four hours we would be landing in Bombay. Alongside the dock we were immediately aware that it had a very different smell compared with Liverpool, and, of course, it was very hot, dusty and noisy. Gazing over the ship's rail we could see lots of the native population, like ants going from place to place, but not so quickly as ants in their nest.

With the gangplanks down, officers came aboard and posted orders. Next morning we were taken to the railway station, again very hot and dusty, milling with people and a smell confined only to India – sweat – and betel nut chewers to carry our kit (though poor ORs packed their own on their backs). We entrained and set off to the unknown, eventually arriving at that famous (some say infamous) camp called Doulali. This was a big tented camp for collection and transit of all ranks both coming and going, covering a vast area.

It was nice to be on dry land. (It took forty-eight hours not to sway on your legs from the motion of the ship). I was called to the Movement Officer and my orders were to proceed to Calcutta, on transport leaving at 0900 hours next morning. I had no idea what this would entail. I was given a railway warrant which was checked at the station in Bombay and I was shown to a two-bunk first-class compartment.

My companion was a Scot and he was very compatible as we talked of his native heath and my experiences there. This was very fortunate as the journey took two days by steam train. There was no restaurant car but a very civilised stop three times a day at a station where meals were served. Again, officers were segregated into the first-class area and served by waiters dressed in immaculate white suits and turbans. We even had starched napkins and *beer*. Life took on a new complexion.

It was fascinating to see the countryside and the local population, despite the flies and heat during the day. At night we had mosquito shutters and lightweight sleeping bags – what luxury compared with the hairy army blankets of the troopship. We arrived at Calcutta only too quickly! I reported to the Movement Officer who informed me that I was posted to the Fort William dental centre, but that at the moment there was no room in the officers' quarters so I would be billeted in Spencers Hotel. Transport arrived and there I was, deposited for the night. The next morning I arrived at last at an army dental centre within the Fort.

It was a joy that I would now be able to do some dentistry. The OIC was the most senior Major in the Dental Corps. He was not interested in promotion, having married a wealthy South African and he lived in the Great Eastern Hotel (the best in Calcutta). When the Japs invaded Burma, he had been in charge of the dental centre at Maymu, twelve miles from Mandalay and a hill station. In the retreat from the Japanese, he and thirty other people decided to walk back to India – communications had broken down, so there were no orders! He buried his valuables and the Mess silver and he and three others survived the walk of some hundreds of miles, living off the country and with the help of the Burmese natives. A well deserved OBE was awarded. Those of you who saw the film *Colonel Blimp*, as portrayed by the great actor Roger Livesey, will have a good idea of the gentleman.

I found that he came from the Midlands and that we had mutual acquaintances. It was a three-officer station, hence a Major as OIC. I well remember him coming to my surgery saying that his tennis elbow was troubling him and asking if I could help with one of his patients. He had broken off the top of a tooth which had refused his forceps-attempted removal. I doubt if in those days there were any dental refresher courses, and after a couple of months, having got to know him well, his tennis elbow became a bit of a joke. He was a member of both the football and cricket clubs and dined me at both of these and at the Great Eastern.

It became almost a pleasure to demonstrate modern dental surgery. One day I found him grubbing around the floor of the office and he was pleased when I offered to help him. He had lost about £1 worth of postage stamps and was worried about balancing his postage book as the Senior Dental Inspecting Officer was due the next morning. He was very pleased when I found them stuck to the bottom of his trousers – he had been sitting on them, sticky side up!

The dreaded visit came the next day – a charming colonel. Everything had been laid on – queues of ORs detailed for dental inspection were dismissed promptly at twelve noon. We all went back to the Mess and later in the afternoon I was told to report to the colonel in the office. After coming smartly to attention a chair was produced and I was told to sit down. The colonel told me that he had read my service record and that he was posting me to Darjeeling (a hill station) to open a new dental centre there.

I would look after army personnel sent there to recuperate from the vicissitudes of war and who had not had leave for a long time. I was overjoyed – my own surgery and my own boss! The other officer there (a rather dour Scot, who was somewhat monosyllabic) was told by the colonel that he was being given an urgent posting to a field ambulance in Burma.

He was to finish his next day's work and to be ready to leave at a moment's notice – I shall never know whether that was deliberate or not. One of his patients, a colonel, had acute toothache in his upper jaw and was advised to have it extracted. The colonel reluctantly agreed. He injected the local anaesthetic and extracted the tooth, then said, "Sorry, sir, I have taken out the wrong tooth. Shall I put it back?" The colonel jumped out of the chair, spitting blood, and he nearly attacked the major, the Scot, who was sent to hospital with 'acute dysentery' (the professional cover-up). He was seen by the psychiatrist and was on the next boat home to his native heath.

Can you guess the consequence? No Darjeeling, and no marvellous posting – Burma, here I come.

The following evening I was transported to Calcutta's Dum Dum airport, having left my tin trunk and clothes at the dental centre. I got aboard a clapped-out Dakota and was airborne. Considering the only experience of flying I had ere this had been with Sir Alan Cobham's flying circus – a 5/- hop around a field – this was quite a new experience. Fortunately there was some comfort, as I was able to lie down amongst the supplies it was carrying.

It wasn't very reassuring, when dawn broke, to see the mountainous region we were flying over, particularly seeing the wings flapping when we dropped a hundred feet, having hit an air pocket. However, when we were later visited by the pilot, he explained that this was quite normal with a Dakota – I was semi-reassured! We eventually landed on a grass airfield near Imphal and gratefully put our feet on terra firma. We were shown to our tents and given a meal of mashed up army rations, but none of us ate much. The plane refuelled and made off on its return trip.

This station was commanded by an RAF officer, an ex-combat pilot. Conditions were very basic. He explained he had not yet had a signal when a plane would be arriving, but after two days of boredom in our tents we learned that it would be there in an hour. The airfield was surrounded by jungle and we had noticed that water buffalo were attracted by the mown grass and were enjoying the grazing. He ordered his jeep a quarter of an hour before the plane's ETA, and his driver took him around the landing strip while he fired his .38 revolver at the animals' feet.

It was certainly effective, but on the return journey it proved disastrous and I had my first battle casualty! He had been holding his revolver on his right thigh, when a bump activated his trigger finger – the bullet grazed the head of his penis and came through the opposite side of his left thigh.

I ignored the minor injury and was concentrating on the copious bleeding of the major wound when the Dakota landed. This was rapidly refuelled, stores and men put aboard, and we were off. I didn't have time to wash my hands and I never knew what happened to him, but what a tragedy for a man who had survived combat duty but not carelessness with water buffaloes.

This plane had just come back from an air drop, so the door was missing. This was the time when the Japs were in steady retreat and their mythical powers had been overcome. The focal point of their lives was to die for their Emperor and so earn eternal Heaven – so said Shintoism.

Back to my second flight. We were, of course, flying over jungle with the same air pockets. No seat this time – an uncomfortable and stressful trip. I learned later that one plane a week was the average loss. (The Japs had been driven back as far as Mandalay). We had just captured the airfield at Schwebo, some twenty miles to the north, and they had regrouped their forces north of Mandalay. Once again I was grateful to put my feet on the ground.

Engineers were working hard to improve the landing strip. Once again I reported to the Movement Officer to be told that I had not finished flying. I was to be taken to a very small aircraft (similar to the LS spotter plane). They were able to land on a strip of grass eighty yards long. I sat on the only seat, behind the pilot, with my bed roll behind me. This time it was an American ex-combat pilot. He was very uplifting when he said, "Jesus, have I got to take you *there*?" This was the final flight for some time. He flew at treetop level, and if it was a high one he just lifted a wing over it. Some thirty minutes later we touched down on the clearing with only a yard to spare.

I got out in a somewhat shattered state. Immediately, stretcher bearers arrived with a body, tipped my seat back, and put the wounded inside. They helped the pilot turn the plane and he waved his hand to me, shouting, "Good luck, pal," and was away with another casualty... To say the least, I was not exactly elated! The stretcher bearers carried my bed roll and this was the way I joined the Second British Division.

I was given a cup of sweet tea, of course with condensed milk. Not ever having liked tea, I started to force it down and even enjoyed doing so, knowing that it was the recommended shock treatment. I was shown to my tent and gratefully lay down on a stretcher to sleep for six hours.

I was awoken with another mug of tea and told to report to the Commanding Officer. Sweaty and with two days' growth of beard, I was relieved to find him in a similar state. He told me that I had joined the Fifth Field Ambulance (code name 76 F.A.). He asked me about my dental experience and if I had dealt with jaw fractures? I replied, "Only theoretically, on the Aldershot course." He said that he was very busy and that a meal had been prepared for me. I was to report back when I had eaten.

On my return he explained the urgency of my posting – the previous dental officer had been performing his morning function over a hole in the ground when a Zero Jap plane had dropped a stick of bombs and he had been killed. He also said that in forty-eight hours the battle to capture Mandalay would begin, that a dead Indian other rank had just been brought in and was in the mortuary tent. It would be a good opportunity for me to wire his jaws and get some practice, before the next live casualties arrived!

I collected my coil of stainless steel wire from the dental equipment, was shown the body, and left to myself. It brought back memories of anatomy days. Fortunately, rigor mortis had not set in and his jaws were still mobile. It was peaceful except for the adjacent noise of battle. You first shape the wire into an eyelet, leaving two strands which you pass through the gums, tighten these securely leaving the eyelet on the cheek sides do the same on the opposite lower jaw, and then thread another piece of wire through the eyelets to lock the jaws together. The upper jaw went well and I naturally became interested in perfecting my technique... Suddenly, there was an intake of breath from the *corpse* – then another... I knew nothing about mouth-to-mouth resuscitation in those days and don't think I would have been interested with his betel-stained teeth. However, I turned him into the life-saving position prescribed in those days and ran out, calling for an MO. His breathing, although slow and shallow, was regular. It turned out that he was a heat stroke case that had been missed amongst all the other casualties. I never knew if he survived...

I, of course, had my leg pulled for my new method of resuscitating the dead! (It is difficult to describe these events to a lay person, but if you weren't somewhat detached, you would have gone nuts and in any case you might be in the mortuary yourself at any time.) From then on the noise of the artillery on both sides increased and a small soldier arrived at my side, said his name was Charlie Finch, that he had been the previous dental officer's batman and could he be mine? Naturally I was only too grateful. There was feverish activity elsewhere. We were only about ten miles west of Mandalay and this was to be the big push to get the Japs on the run.

The gunfire increased overnight and next morning we had an O Group (officers meeting). The CO (I have never met a more sincere, yet analytical man) told us the plan – there would be a frontal attack on Mandalay, and while the Japs were defending this the Second Division was going to do a hook attack to cut off their retreat. Then Five Brigade would start crossing the River Irrawaddy during the night, and if all went well we would be crossing twenty-four hours later at dawn.

The river at our position was at least 300 yards wide and very fast flowing. Next day everything was checked – this was a big

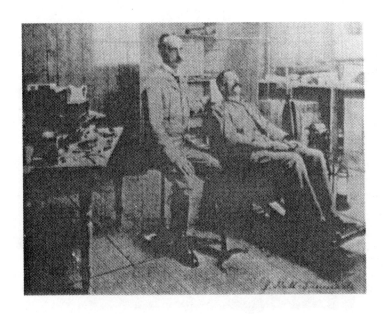

Fig. 1   *Mr Newland Pedley in his surgery - Deelfontein,*
            South Africa, 1900. (top)

Fig. 2   *A Field Dental Unit in operation at No. 10 Casualty*
            Clearing Station, Popperinghe, 1915. (bottom)

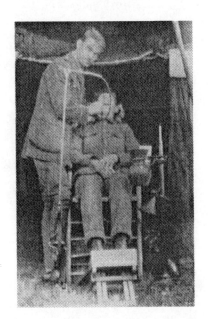

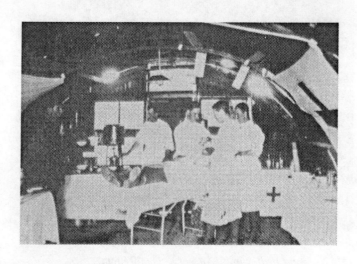

*Fig. 3   An operating theatre of a Field Ambulance in
            action, 1914/1918. (top)*

*Fig. 4   Motorised dental surgery presented to the War effort by the
            Liverpool Corn Exchange, 1917. (bottom)*

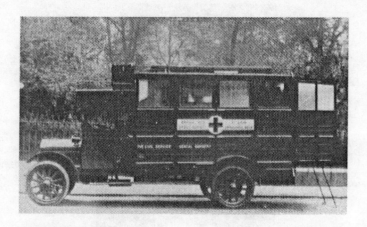

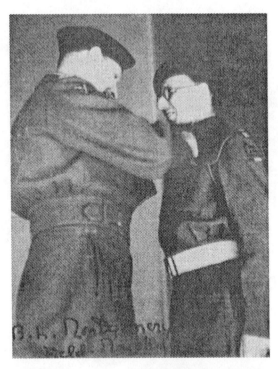

Fig. 5   Capt. B. Hirschfield invested with ribbon of the Military
          Cross by F.M. B. Montgomery July, 1845. (top)

Fig. 6   Capt. D. Glass treating a soldier for a jaw injury during the
          advance through Italy. (bottom)

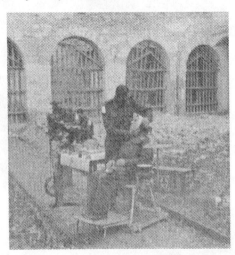

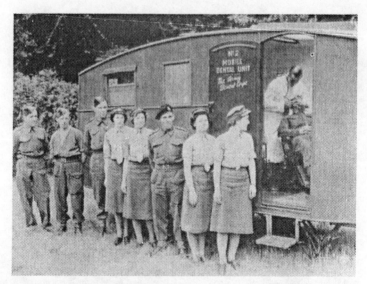

Fig. 7   *A mobile dental unit somewhere in England, 1943. (top)*

Fig. 8   *An 8th Army Field Dental Unit operating in the Western Desert, 1943 (Capt. Attkins, the D.O., later helped to make Himmler's death mask). (bottom)*

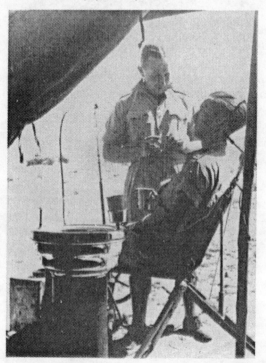

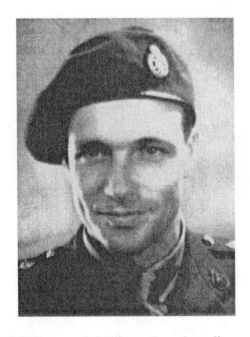

Fig. 9   Capt. D.H. Ridler awarded Military Cross for gallantry in Italy, 1943. (top)

Fig. 10   Somewhere in Burma - a field dental unit. (bottom)

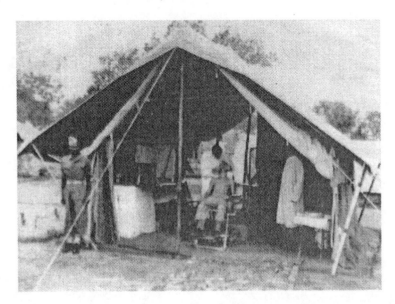

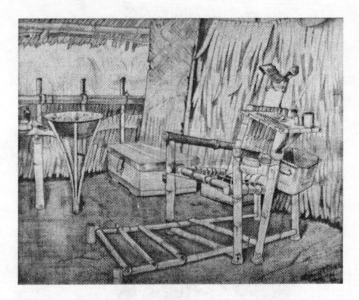

Fig. 11   Chungkai, Thailand - pencil sketch of a dental surgery in the POW Camp constructed from local materials and ingenuity of internees. (top)

Fig. 12   Pencil drawing of a bamboo and string dental chair by Fl. Lt. T. Smith RAF. (bottom)

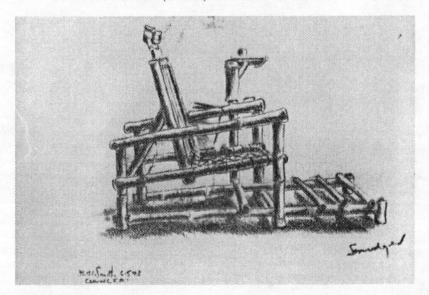

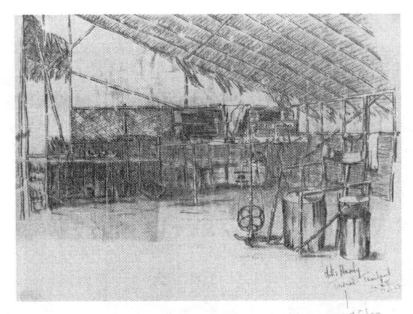

Fig. 13   POW Camp, Tarsau, Thailand, pencil drawing. (top)

*Fig. 14   POW Camp W. F. Finlayson's makeshift surgery, River
        Valley Rd, Singapore. (bottom)*

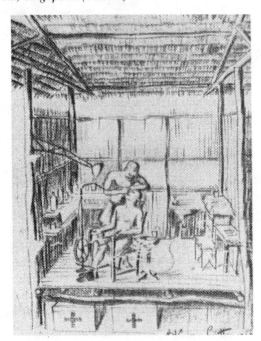

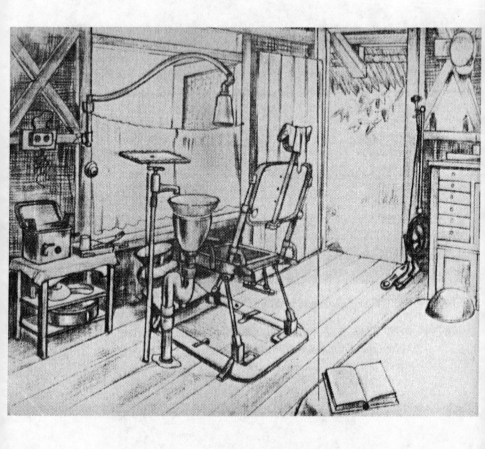

Fig. 15   POW Capt. W. F. Finlayson's makeshift surgery, Kranji, north of the island.

achievement when you think that rafts were made from local trees and canvas pontoons, some of which had been portered down or air dropped. They had to be strong enough to take a three-ton truck. When it was our turn, Charlie Finch came up to me and said he wondered it I would look after the CO's pie-dog, which usually travelled in the armoured ambulance!

This was D-Day+1. The first time a field ambulance had moved into battle so early – certainly in our theatre of war. We made it – the crossing of this fast-flowing river – though, about one-third of the other rafts did not. Some of the canvas pontoons had perished. (There is a sequel later). Strips of white tape had been laid on the ground. MPs were directing us in the right direction according to the colour coding on our vehicles. We carefully proceeded and suddenly realised that we were on our own with no white tapes, and bullets began to hit the ambulance.

The driver, of course, in the presence of an officer, asked for permission to reverse. How he did it on mirrors alone I shall never know, but we found the tapes and arrived where we were to erect our tented hospital, adjacent to the other bank near to the shot-up village of Mingyan, and it was relatively peaceful. I dug out my personal slit-trench – fortunately alongside the river it was sandy – and I must say I lay down in it with my tin hat perched over my face, counting my blessings.

I soon recovered and joined in the feverish activities going on. Where the dog was I shall never know! Within a few hours when we were semi-organised, casualties started to arrive and while the ORs were getting the other tents erected it was all hands to the pump. Even I as a dental officer had to sew up minor wounds and deal with the more serious wounded before passing them on to more competent medics. Mugs of sweet tea with condensed milk were brought to us (I have never drunk tea since!).

The noise was tremendous, but we were very fortunate that no shells landed on us. This went on for forty-eight hours and I have never been so exhausted in my life, after which things calmed down in our little patch and I was able to fall asleep in my trench. Some hours later there was Charlie Finch, shaking me and with a mess tin of hot army rations. I can't remember what it was but it tasted as good as roast beef and two veg. Back to work, doing what I could with the minor casualties, and even able to perform more advanced surgery, which in normal times and without a surgeon's help I would never have contemplated. I don't think some civilian surgeons would have approved!

By D+4 our perimeter had been extended, thanks to the gallant infantry of Five Brigade, not forgetting the Royal Artillery.

An airstrip was cleared, and those little planes started clearing the wounded – things began to ease and get back to semi-normal. We started to get regular meals and by D+5, with five days' growth of board, I actually shaved. Behind my trench, down a steep bank was the river. I slid down the sandy bank, sat on a tiny beach, and said my prayers. It was, of course, very hot. I stripped off and the joy of feeling that water cleansing my body was an experience never to be forgotten. Starkers, I climbed up the bank – the trench had been enlarged to accommodate the Transport Officer besides myself. I stood by it feeling so good, when the Japs' 105s obviously had got our range. I was into the trench and the Transport Officer in on top of me – his boots did me no good at all!

It was a hairy thirty minutes, but fortunately I only had surface wounds on my back, not enough to be sitting on one of the little planes and getting out of this *hell*. We were so fortunate that only one person was killed and we soon heard our own artillery responding. This was the last direct attack on our position. By D+6 the bridgehead had been extended to a couple of miles or so and air drops were coming in.

The next morning the CO asked me to accompany him on a tour of the advanced dressing stations where the casualties were looked after by their Regimental MOs. Unfortunately, we were spotted, but he was an experienced driver who knew by the sound of the shells whether to brake or accelerate! I shall have the utmost respect for him, but we were shattered both mentally and physically.

Just to paint a picture of this time, here is a small diversion... In 1983 I traced his address and wrote to him. Here is an extract from his reply:

> I have the warmest memories of you. The memory sits in my mouth in the unnecessary gap in my eating apparatus. You'll remember at Nagazun, when we had a full complement of patients and were being shelled by those great big horrible things, I came to your tent and said, "For God's sake, Bill, take this tooth out." You looked at me and said, "I can't take it out – it's a normal tooth." "Go on," I said, "I can't stand the shelling and the toothache." You did, and again said,

"It was a normal tooth." My tongue has often wandered to the gap. It just shows how even a brilliant surgeon can be just as stressed as an infantry soldier.

A few days after this we were visited by the Divisional Commander, General Nicholson, and these were his actual words, "I have been a soldier since I was nineteen and have never in all my service seen a medical unit to touch this. To have such a unit functioning so near to the Front is the finest thing for the morale of the fighting soldier that I could wish for. Thank you with all my heart."

This, of course, did exactly what it was meant to do – boost our morale. The fact that the General of Two Division could bother to say those words helped all ranks.

By way of relaxation, I decided to go and see if there were any fish in the river. The bank was about twelve feet high on the bend nearby, so I crawled and put my head over the edge and for half an hour watched a shoal of fish gathered there. Then I was tapped on the shoulder, more work to do. Even so, as usual, it relaxed me. In a Division the medical services are in the charge of an ADMS (Assistant Director of Medical Services), a full colonel.

Next day the CO had a message from him that into our dropping zone a box was to be dropped marked "BLOOD URGENT", and would we guard it carefully until he arrived the next morning. Also we were to let him know if it had been broken in the drop. It arrived safely. He asked Pooh, our CO, for a knife, and we were rather amazed at the amount of packing. When he got to the inside parcel, he paused and said, "Gentlemen, this should be manna from Heaven." It indeed was – twelve bottles of gin. He gave us two, four to be shared by the other two field ambulances, and he and the HQ officers were to have the rest.

He had a friend in SE Asia Command in Calcutta and they had bet on the timing of the recapture of Mandalay, and our colonel had won. He also put us in the picture of how well, after ten days of fierce fighting, the battle was going, indeed within ten days we took what transport we had available and drove to Mandalay. The local population lined the streets and threw us melons which we gratefully cut and gorged on, cheering us all the way. It was a great moment in all our lives.

After viewing the remains of the Fort which had been such a focal point in the battle, we went back to our field ambulance which was still receiving casualties. I was in and out on my little tented surgery depending on the heat of the day. Many of my colleagues will remember a folding canvas dental chair and a foot-pedal drill, but most of the work was emergency extractions.

Another problem was broken dentures, which I had no means of repairing. As they came in they were labelled with the owner's name and number and put in an enamel bowl. The first batch of about half a dozen or so were in pieces, and the next morning they had been gnawed by rats which came from the nearby village, a place still smouldering and full of the stench of bodies. I solved this problem by putting the dentures in an empty metal ammunition box. I discussed the problem with the CO and he sent a request for a vulcaniser, which was dropped together with rubber to repair the plates. This was heated by a meths burner, but unfortunately the meths evaporated in the heat before it was hot enough itself for the vulcaniser to harden the rubber. I had already borrowed a small surgeon's saw to cut the dovetails in the broken dentures, so this was another frustrating moment.

Supplies started coming over the river from the airstrip at Schwebo. Bread was delivered, covered in green mould as it was so long since it had been baked. Nevertheless we tore the loaves to bits and wolfed them. We hadn't heard of Fleming or Penicillin then, but it probably helped with the dysentery which most people had by now, known as 'the squirts'.

Next day we knew we had neighbours, for a local appeared in his dugout canoe from a nearby island. He came to barter for food. Our Lieut. Quartermaster knew a little Burmese and ended up with a half-grown calf in exchange for seventy tins of sardines. One of our RAMC sergeants had been a butcher in civvy street (typical army selection). Naturally the knife was sharp, the animal despatched, hung up in a tree, skinned and jointed. The smell of the cooking made our mouths drip with saliva. Patients and staff slept well.

I went to look at my fish again next day. They were still there, the same shoal. After some thought I cut a bamboo pole, used some dental floss for a line, made a hook from stainless wire, sharpened the point with a file, and with a bit of mouldy bread I was in business. The fact that they had not been fished before was a bonus on my side and in two hours there were enough fish to serve some to our patients, and I was a relaxed man. (I suppose it might have been called 'neglect of duty' and was perhaps the first barbless hook of modern times.)

Of course, as well as the physical wounds, we were dealing with cases of 'shell shock'. The Divisional Psychiatrist visited us, and patients were either evacuated down the line or returned to duty depending on his decision. The RASC transport officer was in charge of the rifles and ammunition that came with these patients, and they were carefully chained and padlocked to a stand. One soldier was to return to duty and while waiting for transport suddenly ran into the ward with his rifle and shot the psychiatrist. His hands must have been shaky as he only grazed the back of his neck. Both were evacuated.

Enough of the battle of Mandalay. We had our marching orders... The rest of Two Division had really got cracking and were moving the Japs back at a reasonable rate. Five Brigade's next task was to move south to the central oilfields of Mektila, go through the other two brigades, and capture a hill fort called Mount Poppa. We set off in our trucks over a dirt track which was the main road... (A little diversion: early on it was found that the Japs had never heard of the Geneva Convention, or they deliberately ignored it. So Red Cross armbands and Red Cross marks on vehicles had to be painted out because they had been prime target for those little yellow bastards.) I had been trained and was expert with a Sten gun, though fortunately I never had to use it, but I wore a .38 revolver in my webbing belt.

We had travelled about fifty miles in the usual heat, refreshing ourselves from the canvas water holders hanging on the outside of the trucks. These cooled by evaporation and were a great boon compared with our water flasks that got so hot. A signal came for us to stop. We could hear gunfire, quite intense but not so near. Then came the order, "Charge your magazines" (i.e. load your guns). A tense moment indeed. However, in half a hour the order came to take the shells out again and to proceed to our next station which was a shot-up monastery on a hill.

The top was flat – whether natural or man-made was not evident – and the remains of the buildings were on one side and the rest was like a barrack square, being quite large. Here we pitched our tented camp. On the north side was a sixteen foot supporting stone wall, and near this the quartermaster and I dug our slit trenches – first

84

priority for everyone. As it turned out, that was the last one I had to dig.

It was about 120°F in the shade, and on exploring we found some monastic cells leading from the basement – obviously they had been used for contemplation out of the heat. Our uniform there was standard; long green denim trousers, stockings and boots, no shirt but a bush hat to keep off the sun and shade your eyes. A long way from the pith helmets and spine pads.

Due to lack of washing facilities either for ourselves or our clothes, we were all covered with sores, ringworm, and so on – you name it, we had it – but our torsos would have been the envy of any modern Adonis disporting himself on the beach, though he might not have envied our slim figures.

Trucks were now able to drive from Schwebo airstrip, so without air drops we had regular food, albeit rather uninteresting rations. It was a marvellously quiet time for recuperation with no casualties pouring in, and I was able to do some routine work. A bright RASC mechanic, realising how hot I got with my foot treadle, rigged up a starter motor run off a twelve volt battery to drive the wheel for the cord and pulley that drove my drill. Our CO in Mandalay was posted back to England – a great loss – but what a marvellous job he had done by his example, for which he later got the OBE. Quite typically he sent us all a letter saying it was for all of us. Everyone worked their utmost in those days, often beyond their normal capacity, and we at last got those bl**dy Japs on the run.

We had all seen (particularly the medical services) what those uncivilised people had done to our troops. One morning we were paraded in the monastery square and told of the next (and last) feature we had to capture – Mount Poppa. I was told that I was to be the advance officer and to arrange for the field ambulance's next move – back to India – to train for our next venture, the capture of Rangoon. I would fly with the Brigade Major from Schwebo next taking key personnel – a Dakota load.

The next day, trucks with supplies arrived and as Q and I sat by our trenches, he calmly told me his surprise news. Of the three field ambulances of Second Division, two had already flown out. Q had taken charge of nearly two years' supply of 'medical comforts' (booze). There were about two thousand bottles of beer, Indian gin, Australia whisky – all caught up because of the lack of road transport and some clerk back in Calcutta doing his quarterly indent of the

Division's entitlement! As our only alcohol had been the occasional tot of rum, this was a serious, though pleasurable, discovery. Q had put this remarkable supply under armed guard. I nearly choked on my cup of tea. He also informed me that we were to have a film show the next day.

I thought that with all the strain he had gone off his rocker, but from his trousers he produced a bottle of gin. I slept very peacefully under my mosquito net that night. The next day, when the film show was announced, you can imagine the cheers. A large white canvas screen was erected quite near to our slit trenches but we positioned ourselves behind this. We could see through the screen even if the artistes were the wrong way around. We didn't want to waste time there as we had a serious job to do...

We were sitting on a high wall looking into our issue pint enamel mugs, contemplating the extract of juniper berry which had possibly been put into the Indian gin. Perhaps foolishly, we did not dilute it with water, but each sip lives on in my memory from all those years ago. After a while, I got more interested in the technical fact of seeing a film inside out, and I turned to Q to remark on this and the fact that all the figures seemed to be in 'doubles', when I found that he was missing ... I looked over the wall and in the half light could see a body at the bottom.

I got a stretcher party and we went around the perimeter at the double (correction, the bearers did and I staggered after them). It was quite a long way round, and by the time I arrived the body was on the stretcher and snoring. I checked him over by torch light and could detect no fractures, only an increased pulse rate. It's said that a drunken man falls into a relaxed state, but this was the first time that I had found this to be true. We tucked him up in bed and I left an orderly to supervise his slumbers, while I did likewise.

Next day he had another problem. He had opened one of the bottles of beer, and before he could pour it into his mug the heat he had caused the golden liquid to squirt out of the bottle. By this time we thought that we ought to inform the CO of the stores. With his superior knowledge we took some bottles of beer to my canvas bath (all of three feet by three feet) in one of the deep monastic cells, filled it with water, and when the three of us met on our nightly tour of inspection our joy was complete – the theory of evaporation through canvas was sustained, and we only lost about a quarter of a bottle on opening.

86

Sod's Law - next morning I was off back to Calcutta. I did hear later that the comforts had been distributed round the brigade and that Mount Poppa had been captured by 268 Independent Brigade. I am sure that this latter was a complete myth. It could not have happened to the glorious Second Division - even Five Brigade.

We took off in the Dakota, all of us very tense and with no safety belts. However, this time there was a door that almost closed. When airborne, we settled down to the long flight to Chittagong. After a few hours, the NZ navigator asked the Brigade Major and myself up to the cockpit. We were flying over the jungle at about 10,000 feet but it was clearly visible. We had already had quite a bumpy ride with turbulence created by the heat.

The pilot was an English officer, again an ex-combat boy - what a good job they did. The plane was set on automatic pilot, and all that was needed was to bring the plane back into a horizontal course by using the driving wheel when we had dropped 100ft or so. We had a natter about what we had been through, and we were invited to sit in the pilot's seat and 'trim' the plane - at least an interesting diversion. We found how heavy handed we were compared with driving a car, and after much laughter and having learned a more delicate touch, we returned half an hour later to the body of the plane to find people puking right and left.

We commiserated with them and lay on the floor ourselves to get some rest. We were grateful to touch down, especially as the pilot had told us that of the a hundred or so flights a week, some two percent, crashed in the jungle.

At Chittagong airstrip we were shown to a concrete shed, which was quite bare except for a wash basin and squatting loos at which we took turns gratefully. Most people just lay on the earth floor to kip (which we had learnt to do on every available occasion). After a couple of hours, I was irritated - not even a cup of char.

I went outside - nice whitewashed stones on the path and a notice to OIC's office. I walked in and found him at his desk. In the best military fashion I gave what I thought was an immaculate salute and tore a strip off him! I told him that it was about time he got off his arse and provided some sustenance for my men who had been fighting their guts out to keep people such as him in a good job for which he was quite obviously incapable.

It was the first time I had torn a strip off a senior officer - his gin-sodden face turned purple. He asked my name, rank and unit, and when he heard my answer he calmed down a bit and began to breathe again! He had actually heard of Two Division and the battle of Mandalay, and within an hour we had tea and blankets to lie on and in two hours a hot meal. By this time, the Brigade Major was woken up and I reported to him what I had done, admittedly with some trepidation. However, he said, "Well done," and went and tore another strip off the colonel.

He also found that we were to entrain next morning for the journey to Calcutta – full circle! This time there were no immaculate servants in white uniforms or stations with restaurants, but dry army rations, and when the wood-burning engine stopped to refuel we were able to make tea from the steam tap. For most of the journey we dozed on our hard wooden seats, but again it was fascinating to see the countryside.

On arrival we were told that we had twenty-four hours before being entrained again to move south and join the rest of the division. The ORs were to sleep in a nearby staging camp, but had we any contacts? We both had! I telephoned my previous CO in Fort William. Had he still got my tin trunk with all my personal possessions? Yes! I said we only had twenty-four hours before leaving for Hyderabad State. It was 9.30 a.m. and I would always be grateful for his reply. There was I, almost as smelly as the beggars in the station or the sacred white cows dropping their dung on the streets outside. "Dear boy, get a taxi to the Great Eastern. I will phone through. My rooms will be at your disposal and I will order your personal requirements."

When I arrived outside this notable hotel, the porter, in his majestic uniform, looked at me as if I was a bit of dirt from the gutter. I mentioned the name of Major Blank and he immediately clapped his hands and I was ushered into the sumptuous suite of rooms. His bearer had already drawn a hot bath and when I was nearly asleep in it in utter contentment, he tapped me on the shoulder and produced an iced *beer*. When I enjoyed this, he dried me with a large white towel and lay me down on the bed, giving me a gentle massage – with coconut oil, I think – but carefully avoiding my open sores. I was then taken back by taxi to the Fort William Dental Centre to pick up my tin box and then back to the station, bearing a mini-hamper of gorgeous food! So... I travelled with the rest of our advanced party to a camp near Secunderbad.

This journey was a mere nine hundred miles, but like the one from Chittagong, it was not exactly first class. The same brewing of char from the engine and the same army compo rations. However, it was quite exciting for the Brigade Major and myself to be back with the rest of the division and the warm welcome we all received.

Next day I was shown the area allocated to the field ambulance, given a drawing of the area and the number of straw huts (bashas). It took three days to plan the reception for when my colleagues arrived. I began to surface and recuperate. The Brigade Officer said next day that he was going to take a truck to Hyderabad and asked if I would like to go. I gratefully accepted.

I had no dental kit until the main party arrived and I was getting bored, though grateful for the lack of battle noises. While he was bartering for and buying fresh vegetables, I was able to take a stroll round a small Indian town, and two hours passed rapidly. I also found a drinks shop and had just enough money to buy a bottle of Parry's 'Naval Gin'. I chose it because of its red seal-like sealing wax instead of a screw top, thinking that if there was any alcohol in it that would have killed off any bacteria.

The camp was, of course, dry. We wondered if anyone knew of our existence. We soon learned that this was because of a security blanket, and rumour had it that we were to do combined ops as soon as Five Brigade arrived to go and capture Rangoon. Within a week my field ambulance arrived and we set about sorting ourselves out. In one basha we made a 'Mess' (i.e. we put our canvas chairs there on the mud floor and hopefully set up a 'bar' where we drank our 'Nibo Panis' – lime juice).

As we expected a move at any moment we only set up a minimum aid station. It was just as well that we had done this, because soon VE Day was announced. This was, of course, greeted with resounding cheers and we could talk of nothing else. Then several three-ton trucks appeared with crates of beer, which were immediately put under guard. There was enough for two bottles per man, and when you take into consideration that there were quite a lot of non-drinkers that was a lot of beer.

After that, we had our evening meal (and even army rations went down well supplemented with fresh fruit). With our appetites whetted by a couple of glasses of beer, we sat down and chatted naturally about Europe and what was happening at home. We all thought that we were the forgotten army and wondered if the Rangoon rumour was true. Our discussion was interrupted by the army phone. The beer and the news had gone to the heads of the members of the Scottish Regiment in our brigade and they were running around setting fire to their straw huts; there were already casualties.

Some officers supervised the setting up of a tented reception ward while others of us set off in trucks and ambulances, grabbing first aid kits and stretcher bearers, throwing their equipment into the now moving transport. We did not need a guide, for the fire was brilliant. (When I look at a casualty on television, I envy them their equipment and facilities).

What had actually happened was that the troops had decided to have a celebration bonfire and the sparks had spread to a straw hut. By the time we arrived, there were four huts blazing, and casualties were being dragged out of the inferno. It was so sad that soldiers who had survived Burma should end up this way and we were more than busy.

My surgery tent was erected and equipment unpacked. My day was a very long one, treating about one thousand patients. My Corporal Dental Orderly became under stress from this and 'saw the Lord'. We were all very grateful for his protection but I had to object to his saying prayers for each patient before I could even say, "Open wide."

The CO soon resolved this problem by putting him in charge of the daily collection of garbage, while I was given one of the theatre orderlies, who was a super assistant once he got to know what was expected of him.

A couple of weeks later we had orders to entrain yet again. Of course we didn't know where we were going, but in actual fact I recognised the countryside – back to Calcutta again, and we ended up in another straw-hutted camp some thirty miles to the north.

We settled down, awaiting further orders, and some of our sores were healing, though some were being reinfected in spite of the use of Gentian Violet, chiefly because our clothes were being washed by the dhobi wallahs in contaminated cold water. It was while we were here that the monsoon broke and it would have made quite an interesting video if such things had been heard of then (maybe Channel Four), as we stripped off and stood in the glorious rain, letting it cool our hot and itching bodies. (I got rid of my ringworm by painting it with concentrated iodine.)

It was while we were here that we heard news of the atom bomb, and fortunately we never had to land on the beaches near Rangoon. This was just as well, for I heard later from our Intelligence Officer that our landing area had proved to be quicksand. The dental chair was a fount of information, a lot of it top secret. Although the atom bomb was a dreadful weapon, it certainly saved thousands of Allied lives – far more than the Japanese casualties; war is always very cruel.

In this camp I had no dental equipment and we were all in a state of limbo. Some eighty percent of the officers had served since 1939, and quite naturally, demobilisation was all they talked about. We had our own transport and all our equipment was stored ready for the next move. The CO, an acting Lieutenant Colonel with whom I did not get on, was such a contrast to Colonel Baker. All he had gone through had made him a martinet – however, I did go in his jeep several times to Calcutta. We had drinks now and in those crazy days drank our gin with cocktail onions and water.

We had a pet chameleon who took over the Mess – fascinating creatures with their slow walk and ability to change colour with the intensity of light. On top of the basha we had lizards and outside at night the croaking of frogs. Some nights through our intoxicated eyes we saw double the number. One night we had an electric storm – the first time I have ever smelt electricity. We never saw our chameleon again.

Orders came through – demob had started – categories one to ten (i.e. the first in were to go home as soon as ships could be provided and this accounted for eighty percent of the field ambulance.)

My order was to report to the ADMS South East Asia Command, next day in Calcutta. I was rather tense as I was driven to his office wondering what had caught up with me, but he could not have been nicer (as I have always found with senior officers). A British Commonwealth Division was being formed to represent us in the occupation of Japan. Five Brigade of the Second Division was to be the British Brigade, and there was to be a combined Australian and New Zealand Brigade plus an Indian Brigade.

He kindly said that my records showed that I was a capable officer in addition to my dental work, and asked if I would be interested in taking charge of all the field ambulance's equipment to Bombay, together with all the other non-demob personnel, and help to raise a new field ambulance for this project? I could, of course, be in charge of a dental centre in India, which would mean promotion to Major, but he would appreciate it if I would accept the former posting with the shortage of experienced officers.

I did not have much time to consider, but my allegiance was very firm to the Second Division and I was not a little flattered that for the first time in my army life I was being given a choice. I said, "Yes, please, sir," and was told that my orders had been typed out and that I could collect them from Major Blank's office. I rose, put on my hat, and gave him my smartest salute, and as I was about to leave he said with a twinkle in his eye, "You will also find that you will be acting Major." (When promoted, you have a six month period before the rank is made permanent.)

I collected my orders and sat down to read them. In two days' time I was to take all non-demob troops together with the equipment to Bombay. Three trucks would be provided and each was to have an armed guard day and night. (There had already been pilfering of army equipment in our relaxed state by anyone who could make a rupee or two). On arrival, we would be met and the equipment would be taken to safe storage. I was to obtain a signature for this, and when it had been completed, transport would be available to take all ranks to a leave camp north of Bombay-Juhu, where we would have five days' leave.

Transport would then take us to Nazik, one hundred and twenty miles north of Bombay, where I would receive further orders. So another full circle Calcutta to Bombay, another troop train and another two day journey, in contrast again to the first one as a gentleman! Arrival at the goods yard, the smell of which was indescribable – no beggars, just rotting humanity lying where it could, and of course the sacred cows. We could not allow our valuable equipment to fall into native hands or we would have lost it, so I ripped off my tunic and helped our faithful ORs to unload the large luggage vans into three-ton trucks. Halfway through this arduous and sweaty work, I called a halt and a char wallah provided mugs of tea – good progress had been made.

As I was sipping mine, a little Indian boy came up to me and said, "You like my little sister, Sahib – two rupees? Will put clean straw under wagon." In other words, I could have had her for about 1/6d old money *with* clean straw! You can imagine the roar of laughter from my troops – the newly-appointed Major being selected for this offer. As I didn't wear any insignia of rank on my deeply-bronzed shoulder I can only assume it was my rather long and straggly ginger moustache which was the attraction. The laughter gave us renewed energy and we eventually saw all our equipment away under guard.

Our own transport arrived and we were driven away to the rest camp on the edge of the Indian Ocean. Straw bashas again, two-bedded ones for the officers. I was shown mine and thankfully sank on to the string bed of the good old wooden charpoy and I lay listening to the sea. I thanked God for His mercy in seeing me through the trauma of these war years...

Just as dawn was breaking, I had a nightmare – the Japs were at me, I was in unarmed combat. I was dealt a severe blow which woke me and I found myself on the floor. The ropes of the bed were rotten and had broken, and I was mixed up with these and the wooden frame. Having extracted myself, I put on my filthy shorts and went for a swim, which cleaned my body and my shorts and cleared the mental strain. I walked up the beach and went to sleep in the shade under a palm tree. Five days of bliss followed before I was summoned to the Camp Commandant.

We were to report at 08.00 to leave at 08.20, so we packed that night, and next morning I found that I was to take my merry band to Nazic (Gandhi's birthplace) some hundred miles north of Bombay. On arrival there, very hot and dusty, we found at least some tents, a flat surface, running water and charpoys. We had emergency rations with us so it was the usual formula – find some wood and brew a char. I read my orders more carefully.

The new Five Field Ambulance was to be formed at this camp and I was to treat the matter as urgent, survey the camp, and make provisional plans for the arrival of a full complement of officers and men. An RAMC Lieut Quartermaster would arrive in the next few days to help me. Together with the newly-formed Five Brigade, we were to occupy Japan, and we should arrive in October for this duty.

Early next morning with my Orderly Sergeant we walked the camp. It had been occupied by Indian troops, whose hygiene had not been of the first order. Filth everywhere – the buckets under the 'thunderboxes' were full, and flies and rats were everywhere. This is a polite description. I was thinking of asking for transport to Nazic to get some native labour, but I need not have worried. The bush telegraph had gone round, led by the local babu.

I negotiated for sweepers, the poorest of the poor, untouchables, and after a lot of haggling, much to the pleasure of all of us, after a few days and many bonfires we had transformed the place. Joy of joys – the quartermaster arrived, a Lieutenant Betteridge, and he took a great load off my shoulders. Everything seemed to happen at once. A transport officer, Ronnie, arrived with a fleet of transport, officers, other ranks, and a new commanding officer to whom I made my report: an Irish RAMC officer, which meant that I reverted to Captain as that was the establishment for a dental officer in a field ambulance. Thus ended my moment of promotion, but I was glad of my Major's pay when I had my next payslip.

The other two captains were both from the European campaign – Ian Troupe and Major Johnstone. So the three of us with battle experience were soon exchanging tales and we became very good friends. The CO made me sports officer and I was to give him a confidential report on each officer after having chatted them up on arrival.

I was able to set up my tented dental centre at last and do some proper work. What a change from the previous months, which had all been administration in its broadest sense. I have never worked harder – trying to make three battalions and Brigade HQ dentally fit for posting to Japan. Everybody was working flat out. More troops arrived. The RASC were responsible for all arms, and of course we did not know what to expect when we arrived in Japan.

I vividly remember two occasions when I had to report to the CO. I had been asked what I thought of Lt Blank. The previous evening I had stripped to my underpants and strolled round to his tent to chat him up. He had recently arrived from England and was worried that his charpoy was not clean. I welcomed him to the field ambulance and sat on his recently cleaned bed. The sun was just going down and, quite frankly, I was buggered, having seen and treated some fifty patients that day. "I object to your sitting on my clean bed in your filthy underpants," he said. He was posted to the North West Frontier, to do what I know not!

On the second occasion the CO told me that in addition to my confidential reports I was to train the RASC in armed guard drill so that we should be able to guard wherever we were in Japan. When I protested that I knew nothing of this drill, he replied, "But you have just been to Burma." I was reasonably competent with a Sten gun and a revolver, but to mount guard was beyond me. He passed me a drill book and I had no option but to salute and say, "Yes, sir," but when I was outside I said to myself, "God Almighty." (I hope the dear Lord forgave me!)

Officer's tents comfortably held four beds, and after the evening meal I lay there, and by the light of a hurricane lamp I digested the manual, before informing the RASC what they had got to learn. My reading was often interrupted by two inch flying beetles banging into the lamp which attracted them. They didn't bother me much because as soon as they hit the floor the rats came in to tidy them up.

Q came to my aid and demonstrated the old .303 rifle. Under his watchful eye he made me strip it down, clean it, and put it together again – lesson one. He also said there was a RASC corporal who had some knowledge in this subject, so I very gratefully ordered him to report to me and together we worked out the drill. We were soon practising with some six other men. When I was reasonably satisfied with them (using, of course, unloaded rifles), I told the CO that we were ready for inspection.

The great day came... We had a lot of rain and the patch on which we were to perform this ritual was, to say the least, somewhat slippery. There was I, some five yards in front of my stalwart six. I followed the book. I gave the order "for inspection port arms", which meant marching towards them and halting to look down the rifle barrels to see if they were clean. Having satisfied myself that all was in order, I brought them down to the attention.

Next, before dismissing them, I was due to do a right about turn, march back five paces and another about turn. I was feeling pleased with myself at completing a complicated manoeuvre (me, a humble dentist), and no doubt this was my undoing. On my second about turn I fell arse over elbow, much to the amusement of everyone watching. It was very good for the morale of all concerned. After more practice we became reasonably competent, and fortunately I never had to use my recently acquired skill in Japan.

A trained RASC officer arrived. The days passed and a 21/C arrived – a Czechoslovakian Major with a good record in the Middle East. We could not understand how he got the posting when we were supposed to be showing the British flag in Japan. After a few weeks this feeling came to a head, and one night after having dined well the QM produced a .303 and several of us took buckets of water and attacked the tent he was sleeping in. The water was thrown over him and several rifle shots went through the roof of his tent.

Full marks to the Czech. He did not complain and we were on much better terms thereafter. We did have a signal next morning from First Camerons suggesting that the next time we had rifle practice at 1.00 a.m. they would like notice.

The days dragged by. Having trained a football team, I took them for an important match against a New Zealand Team and when I returned I found my tent had burned down. My batman had been warming up some water on a primus stove ready for my return and had upset the fuel.

With the long delay in leaving for Japan, leave was arranged in Bombay. We had a four-bedded flat. Max Johnstone and I were in semi-duty, the brothel area was in Grant Road, and number seven was officers only and run by a Madame Andre. It was our duty to visit this house to see if any of our officers there needed treatment in the future. Having dined well at the Taj Mahal, we went in our official transport, to perform our evening duty. We, of course, took off our RAMC and AD Corps badges.

Madame Andre was very co-operative – she prided herself on her 'clean girls'. We sat there having our drinks, a very pleasant duty, but one night she came to us rather worried. She had an RAMC major in her room who was sicking up – could we come? We were only just in time – he was choking on his own vomit. Having dealt with him, we decided that we had better take him back to our flat. He was paralytically drunk and we laid him on the floor. He was in khaki uniform, which meant that he had only just arrived in India, and we proceeded to strip this off only to find that he was wearing woollen combinations underneath!

Thinking that he must be cold, we pulled down the curtains from the tall window, wrapped him in them and flaked out on our beds. Next morning, seeing the body, I had a sudden panic and woke Max. All was well! We arranged for him to be escorted back to his camp. What a fool! He had the equivalent of sixty pounds in his pocket and could easily have had his throat cut for less than that. I heard a nice little story about the madame later, be it true or not.

During the war there was a 'Buy a Spitfire' appeal for collections or donations to make up the cost of £5,000 old money. After the war ended the Governor of Bombay decided to throw a party. He asked one of his staff to draw up a list of residents who had made contributions to the war effort. This was done and invitations were sent out. The great social occasion arrived and, much to the horror of some of the guests, who should be there but Madame Andre. She had bought two Spitfires!

Soon after this, we celebrated Christmas, and then the dull routine went on, relieved by a visit to the officers club at Doulali, which had a swimming pool – pure joy.

In mid-January, the order came for the whole brigade to be vaccinated against plague – a mammoth task to complete all two jabs, and I hope it does not have to be given again as it knocked one out for at least forty-eight hours and we had several near deaths. I suppose the powers that be were worried about conditions we might find in Japan. Soon after this we had our sailing date from Bombay. I remember the invitation from the Dorset Officers' Mess, printed and headed, "Exercise Grapeshot. You will report at 1800 hours and be met personally."

This proved true. When we arrived, we were given a mug of a very strong gin-based cocktail and after an hour we were singing – both regimental songs and some that would not have disgraced the local rugby club! I noticed the brigadier disappear through the flaps of the tent. I thought he had found it too much, but not a bit of it. He came back in his jeep, drove straight into the middle of the tent, with people jumping out of his way. He had brought further supplies of gin! It was some party!

Remember, we did not know what we should find when we got to Japan. We embarked on the Union Castle line's *Arundel Castle*. This was pure joy compared with a troopship and a wonderful cruise was enjoyed by all. I even had a dental surgery. The officers and crew had not had any dental treatment for a long time and I was able to put their mouths in order during this long trip. I was rewarded by being invited to join the officers for a beer each evening.

The Engineer Officer used to bring a bucket of iced brine so we were able to enjoy iced beer – very acceptable in the heat. This, of course, was a professional secret as the rest of the ship was dry until we got to Singapore.

Having arrived there and anchored in the Roads, the good news came that the ban on alcohol was to be lifted, and we could order a case of whisky which would stay in bond until we arrived in Japan. We got this duty free at 12s/6d a bottle. I am sure the ship went down below the plimsoll line when we sailed, though of course we had also taken on water and been revictualled!

At the end of March we approached the Japanese coastline. It was interesting to see land – small coastal plains backed by mini-mountains covered with pine forests. Rice fields on the plains and terraced up the hills as far as they could go. On a pleasant spring day we sailed past island after island, eventually tying up at Kure, the southernmost port of Honshu (the main island).

A wonderful bit of navigation. All was hustle and bustle and we had to stir ourselves after the lethargy that had set in after six weeks at sea. The field ambulance quarters had been a Japanese army barracks, not tents this time, but wooden, built as were a lot of Japanese houses because of the availability of trees and were, compared with Nazic, very clean.

We were soon organised, including armed guards on the gates and patrolling the perimeter (just in case). The best feature was the bath house, in the centre of which was a wooden tub, some twenty feet by ten feet and four feet high. It had bench seats inside and a very adequate supply of hot water. Every evening we sat enjoying its warmth – and our duty free whisky. The top of the tub was wide enough to put our glasses on. Cherry blossom time.

Kure is about fifty miles from Hiroshima and we were naturally interested to see what the atom bomb had done, so one day several of us set off in our own transport to go there. The devastation was *vast*, and we walked around looking at the remains. I had not known that there were any Christians in Japan, but among the ruins was that of a Christian church. Just one wall was still standing and the remarkable thing was that on that wall was a plaque with the Lord's Prayer still intact. It made me say a thank you that I had survived so far in my life. I picked up a piece of pottery which had been fused by the intense heat with other bits of glass and rock, and this I still have.

Later in Kure we had a very sad incident. One of the guards had been cleaning his rifle and despite the well-drilled orders for this he had left a bullet in the magazine and shot and killed one of his neighbours. After the Court of Enquiry we had a military funeral, which, had it not been such a sad occasion, would have made humorous viewing, with us attempting the slow march. However, we did not have any onlookers and we all did our best, including a trumpeter who played the Last Post somewhat off-key.

Orders came through next that Five Brigade were to occupy the nearby island of Shikou. This entailed driving to the ferry to cross to the island. I was detailed to accompany the Second Battalion Royal

Welsh Fusiliers and set up a dental centre in Tokushima. Once again we used wooden army barracks and we were reasonably comfortable, though no mod cons like at Kure. Water for washing was in a wooden bucket, but at least we were dry and warm.

It was now early summer. My dental centre was in a small wooden hut and I had a Japanese interpreter who had been with the P&O shipping line in Yokohama before the war. With his help I commandeered a barber's chair, so not only were my patients more comfortable but so was I.

When you think of the position I worked in compared with modern low-seated dentistry, it's no wonder I have a bad back.

Tokishima had suffered from American fire bomb raids, and as the houses were nearly all made of wood, the devastation was great. It was little different from Hiroshima. The houses are wooden because earthquakes are fairly common, and you are more likely to survive in them than if the house is made of concrete. Also there is plenty of wood available. The Royal Welsh Fusiliers sent patrols to look for any subversible people and found quite a few who were opposed to our occupation and still loyal to the Emperor.

We had Japanese girls to look after us instead of batmen, and it was a bit strange after they had brought your cup of tea in the morning for them to come and help you dress! They even tucked in your shirt tails but this probably shows their different attitude to sex! Their bath houses are communal and no bathing costumes are worn!

The daily grind went on. On one occasion, when it was very hot and humid, I was wearing nothing but an operating gown, bent over my patient, when a F.A.N.Y. breezed in... Shikou is about as big as Wales and there were only two of these girls on the island to look after troops of Five Brigade and their family troubles. I have never seen a more embarrassed female when she viewed my bare bottom!

Autumn came and with it frost, and I was issued with a Valor stove to keep my surgery warm. I was a most popular member of the Mess because I took it back with me in the evening to warm us all up. I'll remind you again that we were all young and had survived the war. On Mess nights the drink was rice beer and there was a tradition of the 'Upside Down Club'. You had to stand on your head with two sponsors to hold your legs, and then in this position you had to drink a pint of beer. I only managed it once!

The colonel was Ap Rhys Price, a marvellous person and a great leader. We were some two miles outside the town and the only concrete building there had been commandeered as a leave hostel, and there were two F.A.N.Y.s there to sort out the troop's problems. We had a typhoon warning and Capt. Bob Davies and I were sent to look after these girls. We did the best we could to batten down all the doors and windows. The girls cooked us a marvellous meal from available rations and also plied us with some of their whisky ration. It was the best typhoon I have ever experienced, although the damage outside was considerable and the subsequent tidal wave also caused a lot of damage.

With the colonel and an escort we made several trips into the surrounding countryside. It was interesting seeing the method of agriculture and the Shinto shrines. Japan is a country of little plains and many mountains. It was not so funny to smell the 'night soil'. "Beware the honey buckets," was the cry.

The Second Royal Welsh Fusiliers were to show the flag and troop their colours in front of the Emperor's palace. A goat was obtained to lead the parade! The great day arrived some three weeks later, and after much rehearsing on the barrack square, the battalion set off for Tokyo. I also was ordered to proceed to Tokyo.

I crossed by ferry to the mainland and took a train for the three hundred mile journey. I was not armed, but almost wished I had been for the Japanese were not exactly hospitable. However, I arrived in Tokyo safely and went to Empire House, a seven storey store specially built of concrete to withstand earthquakes, which had been commandeered for the use of British commonwealth troops.

My dental centre and the Mess were at the top of the building and our sleeping quarters one floor down. It felt quite luxurious to live and work in such a building. I had a Australian orderly as a chairside assistant and we became very friendly. Quite early on we had a problem – the anaesthetic in those days came in a bottle with a rubber cap. You wiped the cap with alcohol and inserted a needle tip of the syringe into this. The ones we had were useless – they came from India, and I think the contents of the bottles had been substituted with water. The dental officer in charge of us was also Australian and when I told him my problem he arranged to have some local anaesthetic sent over from his country. With a supply of lignocaine tablets which you had to mix with sterile water I was able to perform painless dentistry. So, there I was, walking in the streets of Tokyo, the Union Jack on my shoulders, service ribbons on my jacket, a mere captain's three pips on my shoulders, and Americans (from the

Pacific Islands campaign who far outnumbered the Commonwealth troops there) saluting me. They must have thought I was a three-star General!

I had a very interesting lot of patients. In addition to the RWF I had to look after everyone connected with the Commonwealth occupation force. In our old Embassy was the UK Political Liaison Committee (PLC) HQ. Then came the judges to try the war criminals. I met socially the CO of the Eighth Army stockade which was where the Japanese war criminals were held in the Sugamo Prison. He invited me to dine in their Mess several times, and a special occasion I remember was the Thanksgiving Dinner. I took one of the few remaining bottles of Black and White whisky and presented it to the Mess. It was ceremoniously poured into glasses and I only just prevented mine being diluted with Coca Cola! You can imagine how I felt about this precious fluid being drowned in such a way. I survived this incident and had a marvellous meal. Another time there was a party given by the UK PLC. There I first met my Australian CO. It went on for several hours and I was, to say the least, very alcoholic by the time I got back to Empire House and gratefully flaked out on my bed. I couldn't understand why there were bits of glass all over my blanket next morning. Like all stores there were lamps hanging from the ceiling. While I had been asleep there had been an earthquake and the lamps had hit the ceiling like pendulums. Back in Shikou there were gaps a yard wide in the roads. I was lucky to have been in Tokyo.

I became very friendly with the Australian MO, Bob Burston, who looked after all the staff at Empire House. We both enjoyed our evening glass, which was still mostly rice beer – not the most exciting of fluids. Spirits came in once a month with other supplies from Australia. Towards the end of one month, stocks were very low, and there was only a bottle of Cherry Brandy and one of Advocaat on the shelf. Bob and I decided to drink a mixture of the two, and ever afterwards we were known by our fellow officers as 'Blood and Pus'.

On one occasion we were invited to the Russian Embassy. We were warned that they would want to drink us under the table, and being British we were not going to let this happen. We were on our friendliest and best behaviour, and fortunately they had potted plants which we used to pour our drinks into after embracing our comrades. We left them lying on the floor and walked back to Empire House. Another social occasion was the combined British, Australian, New

Zealand and American Officers' dance. I had got quite friendly with an American nurse who accepted my invitation to the dance.

It was quite an occasion – a buffet supper and an American jazz band. It went with a swing. I introduced my girlfriend to my brigadier and lost her for a couple of dances. When I returned from the buffet, they were sitting on a couch – he with his hand down the top of her dress. This irritated me so much that for only the second time in my army life I tore a strip off a senior officer. He realised that he had been carried away with drink and even apologised the next day! Came the end of 1946 and a marvellous Christmas dinner, the menu of which I still have.

Soon after, I was posted back to Shikou, with the Second RWF. I had not been back there long before orders came through for Five Brigade to go to Malaya. Once again, I was to be the advance officer of Five Field Ambulance. I arrived at Kure with my other ranks. only to find that our troop ship was to be the *Dilwara*! How strange to meet up with her again. I reported to OC troops, and after chatting he said that he would like to see Hiroshima and asked if I would be prepared to take his place for forty-eight hours and supervise the troops coming aboard, to which I agreed. Strange, the variety of jobs other than dentistry I had to do at this period in my life. However, we set off for Singapore and as I had accommodated the OC troops I had no duties during the whole of the trip! With no dental centre on board it was a very nice cruise as far as I was concerned.

We were taken to a camp north of Singapore in the state of Johore Baru, where we still had nothing to do. There was a nine-hole golf course nearby and although most of us had never played before, we knocked a ball around. We then went to the Club House for a round or two and played poker dice. I still have my favourite number five iron which I won from a major due to my skill in lying about dice in my hand. Max Johnstone had a relative up country who was a rubber planter and he invited us for a weekend's shooting on the edge of the jungle beside his estate.

We were able to order a fifteen cwt truck to take us a hundred and fifty miles. Max had not seen his relative for some years, so it was quite a party. We were taken round the estate and shown the art of tapping the trees, then we had a light meal to prepare us for night shooting on the jungle borders. We were after mouse deer – a miniature deer about nineteen inches high – and we wore battery-operated lights strapped to our foreheads like miners' lamps.

The scheme was to stalk an animal and pick up its eyes in the beam, then switch off and stalk nearer, switch on again to pick up the eyes, aim at them and shoot. I followed the instructions, and when I got near enough to the eyes I let fly. I saw the animal fall, and it was with some pride that I went to pick up the body only to find that it was a big bull frog! However, other members had more success and my shooting episode caused a lot of laughter round the brigade when we returned.

After a few more weeks, it was decided that Five Brigade would be disbanded and reformed in the UK. The remainder would become Five Independent Brigade. So that was the end of my wonderful association with the Second British Division. The comradeship and loyal support of every man was one of those remarkable things about the war. The Second British Division was no more remarkable than any other, but all of us who served with it had something above the ordinary relationship of man to man.

A posting came through. I was to be posted to the British Military Hospital in Singapore and take over its Dental Centre. Thus, routine work once more, until one day the Chief Surgeon came and said he had a jaw fracture case and would I come and look at the patient with him. Compared with some of the wartime fractures, it was relatively simple. So next morning I was with him at the operating table, scrubbed up and with rubber gloves on. I found that the gloves were being worn through by the stainless steel wire when I tied the eyelets I had made through the gums. So I ended up throwing the gloves on the floor. However, a successful operation was completed.

One vivid recollection I have was that of the quartermaster whose room I shared – two beds with mosquito nets above them. He was an alcoholic and had two raw eggs with a dash of Worcester Sauce for breakfast. We had a Mess party one night and retired rather late. I always put my notecase under my pillow, but on this occasion the whole Mess had been done over by thieves. It had gone, like everyone else's. Weeks went by and then a phone call from ADMS Singapore.

"What time do you get up, Edmonds?"

"6.30, sir."

"Right, report to my office at 7.30 tomorrow. I have arranged transport for you."

I wondered what might have caught up with me and arrived at his office in some trepidation on the dot next morning. After the traditional salute he told me to sit down and said I was to go and inspect Number Twenty-One and Twenty-Two Dental Centres at Tanglin Barracks at GHQ Singapore. He was worried by reports he had received and gave me written orders to this effect. It is rather embarrassing to go through fellow professionals' activities, but in the army you have to carry out orders. Apart from the unconventional way the centre was being run I found a bottle of potassium cyanide containing sixteen ounces of this lethal stuff in an unlocked cupboard. This had probably been left by the Japanese. I took my written report next day, including this final piece of information. The expression on his face would have made a good Bateman cartoon. I was posted Officer in Charge of the GHQ Dental Centres.

I was treating all kinds of patients from ORs to generals of SE Asia Command, civilians from the Embassy and Immigration Officers. One of my patients was the Senior Movements Officer in control of all the port shipping. Nobody wanted to take on the sixteen ounces of potassium cyanide, so he and I decided to put it in an ammunition box, load it with bricks, and take it out into the Roads of Singapore and sink it. Next Sunday morning off we went and cast it overboard – it didn't sink! I had visions of it being washed up on a shore and local inhabitants exploring the contents. Providentially, he had an armed guard with him who put some gun shots through it. We were very grateful to see the bubbles rising, but I wonder what happened to the fish!

This was about March 1947. My demobilisation number had come up and I was looking forward to returning to the UK, but I was told that it was essential for me to carry on in my appointment until a suitable replacement had been found. Compared with what I had been through, life was very good. I was enjoying a day's work and even power cuts did not interfere. I asked for and was given a Singaporean boy who used to pedal the treadle drill when the cuts occurred so that work was not interrupted. The Senior MO looking after the personnel GHQ had a staff car. I soon became friendly with him, so on Sunday mornings we proceeded to the Royal Singapore Swimming Club, swam a few leisurely lengths, and then had breakfast – a luxurious event sitting under an umbrella served by waiters in their immaculate white uniforms – with starched napkins and a traditional English breakfast. The alternative to the Mess Dinner was to go into Singapore, where there were many restaurants. Soon after I arrived I went to one of these and ordered steak and chips. Having finished this, to the utter amazement of the waiter, I ordered another steak, which went down very well! It was such a delight after all the army rations. Another side of my life was to go into St Andrew's Cathedral and just sit in peace and quiet, and while there I would thank God for keeping me alive.

The climate of Singapore is very hot and sticky, ninety degrees Fahrenheit and ninety percent humid. I took up golf as a relaxing sport. A group of us played once a week, wearing shorts and sleeveless shirts, with towels tucked into our shorts, and we had Malaysian boys to carry our clubs. On one occasion I addressed the ball on the first tee and had forgotten to wipe my hands on the towel. The club went up into the top of a nearby tree and the ball was undisturbed! The boy shinned up the tree, recovered the club and the game continued!

I was informed at last that a replacement officer was on his way and I was, of course, elated. Then two things happened. First, Tony Roach, the immigration officer (whose teeth I had sorted out) came to see me and asked if I would be prepared to stay in Singapore. As there was no European dentist there he would arrange for me to have a government grant to set up in practice there. Second, I was ordered to report to the ADMS South East Asia command who said that he had looked at my army records and was offering me a regular commission.

I think I did the right thing at this time in refusing both offers. If I had accepted the first with all the drinking parties necessary to keep 'in the swim', I would probably not be alive now. If I had become a regular officer, I would not have met my dear wife, who has typed these memoirs.

My turn to return home came and it was arranged for me to board HMS *Glory*, a light fleet aircraft carrier. She had been to Australia at the end of the war to show the flag. How lucky I was – only a fortnight to go before I was to be on my way home, and then not on a troop ship but as a guest of the Royal Navy.

My countdown started, and at the beginning of the last week I started handing over the dental centre with all books and records up to date. Then, I received a phone call from General Commanding Medical Services SE Asia. He would like some spare dentures before I left. When I examined his mouth and dentures, he said he wanted the spare ones to match his existing set (i.e. he wanted the new bottom denture to match the existing upper denture and vice versa!)

This is a very difficult technical procedure. My mechanics were wonderful, one even worked through the night, and at 9.00 a.m. when I was due to board the aircraft carrier I fitted the general's new dentures. I often wonder what he put on my officer's record but I was away to the Naval Base on the Northern part of Singapore Island and I couldn't have cared less then.

As I walked up the gang plank I wondered if it was really true that here I was, a 'brown job', going aboard a naval vessel for my return home.

Nothing could have been nicer. They were expecting me and made me feel very much at home. My baggage roll and tin trunk were stowed away by a steward, and within two hours we had left Singapore Island. What a treat! Nothing to do except enjoy the voyage. Being a ship of some twelve thousand tons, there was a dental officer on board. I was introduced to him and we discussed our various experiences. We sailed on, a lovely voyage, 'jilltying' fish and porpoises, and made land at Trincomalee in Ceylon, which had been a naval base for years. We took on water and supplies and in forty-eight hours we were off again. Several more officers came on board here to return home. One of these had acute toothache, but he took one look at the 'toothy' and said, "Good God, not him again." A plan was made. (When I found out that I could drink as much gin at 2d a nip as the Fleet Air Arm Officer, I was accepted as one of them.) We decided to get the 'toothy' drunk and the officer with the bad toothache likewise. It was surprising how long this took. I had to pretend to have neat gin, but the steward served me with water. When the 'toothy' was paralytic, we put him on his bunk and relieved him of the keys to his surgery, and the patient was lifted up into the dental chair. I went through the motions of inserting some local anaesthetic, though on reflection I don't think it was necessary. However, the next morning the toothy complained of a headache, and we had one naval officer very pleased that he had not got toothache! From then on, I was accepted as one of the boys.

We played deck hockey – quite a different game from the hockey that I had played at the age of fourteen. The ball was a piece of rope curled around to be more like an ice hockey puck. Imagine the deck of an aircraft carrier with no guard rails, and if one didn't stop running in time there was a forty foot drop into the ocean – quite stimulating! There were no planes on board, so we played badminton in the hangar. This became a game of some skill and judgment. If the ship was rolling from side to side, a high drop shot could come into either court, and if it was rolling fore and aft the high shot could come back into your own court.

We sailed on, all looking forward to our demobilisation and civvy street. The evening get-together in the bar was a great time for swapping experiences and speculating on what we thought would happen when we got home.

Eventually we reached Aden and were allowed ashore. This was just before the Suez trouble, and even so you could feel the hostility of the natives – even a camel belched in my face! The smell was indescribable. I've had patients with bad breath, but this was an all time high! Forty-eight hours were enough for us all, but the voyage through the Suez Canal was just as interesting as when I had been going in the other direction. So into the Mediterranean, and on to Malta, where we moored in the harbour and shore leave was allowed. Officers could wear civilian dress – white shirt, denim trousers, and a trilby hat! My memory is a little hazy, but with six friends we proceeded in regulation dress (they had found me a trilby), to explore the town. On the quay we hired horse-drawn carriages to do the famous Gut. This is a steep hill with lots of bars and other diversions of the female variety. By the time we got to the bottom of the street we had already lost a couple of our party. The rest of us were hungry, and as one of the party knew a good restaurant on the north of the island, off we went in our horse-drawn vehicles. We had a sumptuous meal. I was more than a little tired and under the influence of a good deal of drink and so I decided to go back to the carrier. I summoned a carriage and proceeded back to the quay, refreshed by the night air, and trusting the driver as I didn't have a clue where I was. Eventually I recognised the quay, but was worried that the carrier was the wrong way round! We had a few words, and to this day I regret that I refused to pay the driver the fare. When he became abusive, I hit him fair and square on the chin. Eventually I found a little boat to row me back and sank gratefully back into my bunk...

The next morning we heard that there was to be a delay before sailing, as the admiral's car, which we were taking home, had to be washed and polished. It was Sunday and the bars were shut, so we went to a club of which the naval officers were members, and another drinking session followed – this time served by a blonde barmaid who looked like Marilyn Monroe – a good time was had by all. This had to be cut short when we learned that the admiral's car had been put on board and that we were to sail at 4.00 p.m. – back to HMS *Glory*, and grateful for the forty-eight hours, thanks to the car.

As well as our sporting activities, we had some film shows on the hangar deck. Old as they were, they made a very welcome interlude.

On through the Med and we arrived at Gibraltar. No shore leave this time, only a pause to pick up water and stores. On to the Bay of Biscay, which could not have been more clement. Then forty-eight hours before making the English coast, having enjoyed a film show in the evening (a mild one as regards drinking). I walked through one of the four foot watertight doors, caught my head on the top, and finished up as a casualty in the sick bay! It was not a deep wound but fairly extensive on my scalp and needed a dressing secured with plasters! It did not make me look very handsome – and only twenty-four hours from home and demob!

Plymouth, and six of us were to go ashore here. In the first boat to come alongside were the customs' officers, and we were all somewhat apprehensive as we sat at their table answering their questions. I had golf clubs bought in Singapore – "You did say you had had them more than twelve months?" – and so it went on. They were very helpful to those of us who had been a long time abroad. A motor fishing vessel came alongside the gangway and the crew took our luggage. All we had to do was to climb down the precipitous steps... What a moment! After all those weeks we were going to be home in dear old England. We arrived at the quayside at low tide with the quay some eighteen feet above us. There was a dock strike on, so we had to organise ourselves. We found a rope derrick and hauled up our bits and pieces to the quay, but we were not too pleased with this reception after all the years overseas. We found a telephone and ordered taxis to take us to the station. We found a train just about to leave for London and just got our luggage in the guard's van and ourselves on the train as it moved off. There was plenty of room and we left our hand luggage on some seats and made our way to the restaurant car. After all this effort of sorting ourselves out we were really looking forward to some British beer. Never had it tasted so good – Bass at its best! We then had another one! On looking around I saw that several civilian passengers seemed to be staring at me, but I thought it just my imagination. Naturally, the effects of these two bottles had to be dealt with and I made my way to the lavatory. There I looked in the mirror and found that the exertion on the quayside had opened my wound and I had congealed blood down both cheeks!

My face was a dull yellow from the dust so it was no wonder that people were staring at me! At the station I was able to make a change and proceed to the demobilisation centre at Aldershot. What a coincidence that having started there, I was to finish there too.

I was given a brown double-breasted suit, black shoes, and a brown trilby hat. I was able to phone my parents in Birmingham and they drove down to Reading the next morning where we had a happy reunion after all those years. They were naturally worried by my head wound and the yellow colour of my face (from the Mepacrin anti-malaria tablets) but it was a very happy occasion, especially for me to meet my young brother John again.

Father had bought an Austin eighteen horse power seven-seater in 1939 and into this we just had enough room to pile my tin trunk and bed roll and then we drove back home to Somerset Road in Birmingham. What I noticed most was the greenness of the countryside.

Mother, having lived through the First World War, had a vast stock of tinned goodies which she had started buying in 1939, so there was plenty to eat over and above rationed food. Here I have to make a confession – the only thing I did not declare at the customs was a rope of Japanese pearls which I had in the top pocket of my battle dress, firmly buttoned down. Mother was more than pleased to have these among the other presents I had accumulated. She later gave them to Sheila, my wife, who still wears them on suitable occasions.

I had accumulated demobilisation leave of three months on full pay, due to my being unable to take leave on my last posting in Singapore. After the initial emotional celebrations and playing some indifferent golf at Harborne Golf Club, I began to get itchy feet and decided to visit some friends. While with my friends, the vet and his wife in Maidstone, I had a phone call from home telling me that Philip Hughes was also demobbed and was in London. He had rented a flat behind Marble Arch and to this I made haste. It was a somewhat hectic reunion with my great friend from student days and whose best man I had been. After several days of what seemed like riotous living, he said that now he was a married man he wanted to find somewhere to join a practice. A big dental supply firm then acted as agents for the profession, and one afternoon I accompanied him to visit the secretary who ran this office. As he went through the list of available positions I was able to chip in with advice. This was noted by the secretary who asked for my own particulars. I explained that I was not yet interested in work due to my extended leave. However, she telephoned me at the flat the next day to say that it would be worth my while to make an appointment with Mr... at number one, Harley Street! I was due to return home in a couple of days so I fixed an interview and ended up agreeing to become his assistant. (It turned out that I had treated some high-up officers in Singapore who were his patients.)

So back to Brum and a more mundane existence – definitely a more sober one!

After due consideration I wrote to Mr... and said that I did not think that with my love of the country pursuits I could contemplate living in London...

Cotterill and Co, the dental firm, kept sending me lists of vacancies, and amongst these was one at Buckingham House in Malvern. Mother and Father had some farming friends at Hanley Swan, so one day I took Dad to work, picked up Mother, and drove over to the Wilsons. After lunch I decided to phone Messrs Strickland and Godfrey, who suggested that I drop into Buckingham House at 5.30.

The outcome was that I started in practice there on the day after Boxing Day in 1947 and I stayed until retired... Fate moves in a mysterious way!

BRIEF MEMOIRS OF CAPT. T. W. FROST, AD CORPS

T. W. Frost, Captain, Army Dental Corps, volunteered 1939 for active service. First posting to Saxmundham busy with local troops. Had a clinic attached to a schoolhouse.

In January 1940 he was posted to the Thirty-eighth British General Hospital, assembling at Hatfield to await active service overseas. Some temporary service in hospitals around this area. Did a time at East Grinstead, studying the methods of Archie Macindoe.

In January 1941, sailed with the Thirty-Eighth BGH from Gosforth in a large convoy, guarded by HMS *Ramillies* and several destroyers. Landed in Shoubah, Iraq for more temporary duty. Very frustrated, personnel lived in tents in the desert.

Sailed back to Bombay, by train to Poona and more temporary duty. After some weeks, the BGH on the move again to destination Bangalore, Southern India.

In 1942, hospital was set up in barracks, vacated by Cavalry Brigade. Became a first-class working hospital. Time spent getting troops in vast numbers dentally fit. Some private work and a few casualties from Libya. Went on tour for two months.

In March 1944, Thirty-Eighth BGH left Bangalore complete with personnel and equipment for Galaghat, Asram (presumably to be ready for the battle to regain Burma).

Tented hospital set up on hillside during the monsoon, immediately filled with waiting troops and some casualties. Conditions meant everyone consuming at least twenty pints of fluid per day and rather unpleasant fluid at that. Surgery was two thatched basha huts on concrete plinths. No running water and no electricity. Much make and mend! Taking a bath meant standing in the rain.

On 7th August 1944 posting arrived to more forward area, taking Orderly and Mechanic, destination Imphal. Thirty-Eighth British General Hospital began to be split up.

On 7th August 1944 posting arrived to more forward area, taking Orderly and Mechanic, destination Imphal. Thirty-Eighth British General Hospital began to be split up.

Delivered exhausted officer and immediately very busy. "Today I saw seventy patients." There, four mechanics worked in tiny tents, the temperature over 100°F. Primus stoves used for sterilising, bodies were stripped to the waist.

Evidence of fighting all around – fox holes, dug-outs, dead trees, white crosses, all supplies carried in by a constant flow of wounded.

Extract from letter dated 6/11/44:

...This lad stopped the recoil of a 75mm cannon shell with his face, and it didn't do him any good. His right upper jaw was pushed in over to the mid-line, teeth and all. His lower lip was split open vertically in the centre and he had a horizontal split right through just above his chin...

Burrows (anaesthetist) and I spent two hours on him and he looked quite a pretty picture when we'd finished, under regional anaesthesia (with a ¼ morphia) I applied eyelet wires, reduced the fracture completely and tied him up again in correct occlusion. He sutured up his lacerations, cleaned him up, filled in sulphanamide to his wounds and sent him off to Calcutta in two days time.

I have no further records, but as the Battle for Burma became further away from Imphal, sisters and medical staff were posted in all directions.

A MEDAL FOR BURMA
The story of Captain M. A. Freeman, Army Dental Corps, MC.

Following a period of service in various dental centres in Northern Command, I joined the 222 Corps Field Ambulance attached to Corps HQ at Scotch Corner (Catterick). This particular Field Ambulance was a new unit, and I stayed with them for some months until I was sent overseas with a draft of dental officers to India.

The first posting in India was as a dental officer attached to the Third British General Hospital, Poona. For a time this was a pleasant life, little different to that of a peacetime dental officer. However, after a time I was posted as dental officer attached to the Fifth Field Ambulance, Fifth Brigade, Second British Division.

The whole division had recently arrived out East and were undergoing re-equipping and fairly intensive training. This training was primarily in jungle warfare and it then switched to assault landing training for an intended amphibious assault in Arakan. As it transpired, this assault was made by another brigade and not the division as a whole.

The next phase was precipitated by the rapid Japanese advance northwards from Burma into Manipur State. Imphal became completely cut off and Kohima, the last strongpoint before Dimapur the main base, was surrounded. The Second Division was principally the force put in to halt the Japanese advance on Dimapur and to relieve the situation at Kohima.

Up to this time the dental officer had been primarily engaged in securing dental fitness in the personnel of the brigade, but this role now changed. The brigade deployed in a position between the Japanese forces just north of Kohima and the one main road leading to Dimapur, some seventy miles further north.

For a time this was frustrating, as the beleaguered hilltops of Kohima were visible a short distance away, but it was not possible immediately to open up a permanent corridor for relief forces to get in and the garrison to get out, although some casualties were evacuated from the garrison before the enemy 'ring' closed again.

The assault on the Japanese forces investing Kohima was then intensified with 'hooks' to the west and the east. Part of the Fifth Brigade, including part of the Fifth Field Ambulance, did a 'left hook' and eventually captured the Naga Village area – the eastern part of Kohima. Our forces, having got into the Naga Village, the enemy promptly closed the gap and we found ourselves holding a fairly tight perimeter and relying on air drops for all our supplies.

Casualties were fairly heavy, and during this period the dental officer spent his time giving first aid to maxillo-facial injuries, acting as a general casualty dresser and giving intravenous anaesthetics, and so on. It was very difficult to hold casualties in the tight perimeter, and so walking wounded who were no longer effective were evacuated through enemy-held territory by jungle paths.

After some time, the besieging Japanese gave way under the assaults from three sides and what remained of the gallant defenders of Kohima were successfully evacuated. This was the turning point of the Japanese thrust towards India.

After a short time, the Fifth Brigade and the Fifth Field Ambulance formed part of the force given the task of clearing the main road south from Kohima to Imphal. The country was very hilly, with only one main road, and was ideal for road blocks and the establishment of strongpoints by the Japanese rearguard. Most road bridges were 'blown' and bridges were usually covered by an enemy strongpoint, so progress was necessarily slow.

During this time, the dental officer spent his time assisting with general casualties. The Japanese encirclement of Imphal was broken and Fifth Brigade then had a period of rest. Not so the dental officer, who was lent to a casualty clearing station, where there was plenty of work to do.

The advance was then continued south beyond Imphal to Tamu and the Kabau Valley. By this time, the Japanese were in poor physical condition, but they still resisted strongly with the now familiar pattern of 'blown' bridges, road blocks and bunkers built into hillsides.

114

During this time the field ambulance provided a full service to casualties. It was also possible to take in and provide immediate medical and dental aid to long-range penetration groups who had spent long periods in enemy-held territory and had suffered very considerable physical hardships.

At this stage, reminiscence of this field of operation ceases, as I became ill with hepatitis and was evacuated to Imphal. From there I was flown to Comilla, and from Comilla to Calcutta. From Calcutta I travelled the length of India in a hospital train to Secunderabad, where six weeks were spent in hospital.

After a month's recuperation in Darjeeling, I rejoined the Fifth Field Ambulance, which, together with the rest of the Second Division, had been withdrawn in preparation for the final assault on Central Burma. This, however, I did not see, as I was repatriated to the UK.

Before I left the field ambulance, I was delighted to find that my replacement was to be Captain McGlade, whom I knew quite well. It is sad to relate that he was killed very shortly after taking over. Back in the UK, I finished my army days, first at the dental centre attached to the School of Infantry, Warminster, and then for a short time at the Army Dental Centre at my home town, Cambridge, which, strange to say, overlooked my own civilian practice on the other side of the street.

AWARD OF THE MILITARY CROSS – CITATION

Lieutenant (T/Captain) M. Freeman, MC, AD Corps (Burma)
On the 15th May, while conducting Stretcher Bearers down a track, loading from the Kohima Naga village area to the Zubza valley, mortar fire was opened on the party. Captain Freeman might well have taken cover with others, but he immediately attended to the freshly wounded patients and bearers instead, moving from one to another with complete disregard of personal safety while mortar bombs continued to fall on the track. I witnessed Captain Freeman's behaviour on this occasion and undoubtably by his action he prevented further casualties. Captain Freeman is strongly recommended for the award of MC in recognition of his gallant behaviour on 15th May 1944.

THE BATTLE OF KOHIMA

Prologue

The Battle of Kohima in the Naga Hills of Assam in 1944 was an extraordinary event, not like any other in World War Two. In the first battle, one of two, a tiny British Force in a very heroic action, held the key position of Kohima against overwhelming odds for two critical weeks. In the second battle, a British and an Indian Division fought a Japanese Division day and night over a further two months for control of the road running through this mountain village. Nearly all the fighting was savage and at close quarters allowing little respite for either side in action. Even when starving, the Japanese would never surrender. Conditions were atrocious in the very steep, forest-covered terrain. Frequent heavy tropical rain hampered movement, which was already a hazard due to heaps of stinking unburied dead. It was a hard-won victory and very important in the strategy of the war in Burma.

LETTERS FROM BURMA –
1944–45
[Major (Retd) F. D. R. Geldard,
Army Dental Corps]

On the 19th March 1944 the Second Division was told to concentrate ready for a journey of 1,500 miles by air, or 2,000 miles overland. Recently Orde-Wingate had been operating with his Chindits and the Special Force and harassed the Japs. The first of the Division arrived at Dimapore on 1st April 1944 and in early April we, the Fourth Field Ambulance, started on our journey from Bangalore to one of the most beautiful but wet countries on earth. In North Burma one gets up to forty feet of rain as well as sandflies, ticks, mosquitoes, and leeches. General Slim's description was: "No comfort for man or beast in these hellish jungles and mountains."

We left by train, which stopped at meal times and we got out on to the track. The cooks made tea and handed out army biscuits, bully beef and cheese each time. After four days we stopped at a flat dry area where Dakotas were waiting. Fourteen got into each plane sitting on the floor round the sides. Two planes set off together and the American pilots amused themselves and frightened us by flying under each other and generally having games. Eventually we reached Jorhat, an American airfield. When we arrived by truck at the spot as ordered, we were told that we had gone too far and must wait for tanks to pass through. After India this area was quite a contrast – it was very green. The jungle was thick and we settled down on the edge of the road.

Trenches were dug for us to sleep in, and we had a large deep hole with groundsheet covers and a portable electric light set with which to treat casualties. Unfortunately for the casualties and for us, there was a large gun at the side and the firing shook the ground and was deafening. However, we were well guarded by troops from the brigade. I helped with dressing the wounded and could even do emergency dentistry using the instruments that I carried in my pack, otherwise all I had was a bedroll and one change of shirt and slacks. We had sandbags around the surgical trench – bags were easy to fill as the ground was soft and sandy and trenches were easy to dig. Snakes liked the sand bags and the RSM killed two hiding in them. We were now wearing anklets which we hoped would help in the event of a snake striking low. My dental surgery consisted of the patient sitting on a rock with my orderly holding his head. At night we had to be quiet and any talking was done in a whisper. We got up at 4.45 a.m. – it was then rather cold – to be alert at dawn, a time when Jap patrols were active.

My treatment of maxillo-facial injuries consisted of removing any unattached pieces of bone and wiring up with stainless steel wire any parts with some attachment, bones or teeth, rather like a jigsaw puzzle. In my spare time I could watch our planes bombing the Japs in the wooded hills. This was Nagaland, and the Nagas who lived in villages on the hill tops or well up the sides followed us around picking up empty tins and rubbish.

On April 26th, the first heavy rain started and we were given monsoon capes, but we still got very wet. The first night I woke to find myself lying in water; there was a leak between the groundsheets but my mate, still maintaining a sense of humour, said it was not rain! Breakfast at 0630 consisted of porridge, two bits of bacon with bubble and squeak, and one slice of bread with marmalade – supplies were still quite reasonable. The Japs were now only one mile away and I could watch the seventy-five millimetres, the mortars, and the Bren guns firing away from a hill. All we could do now was wash our hands and faces, our clothes remaining unchanged for days. In May, things improved somewhat as we had little bivouac tents with netting at the ends to cover our holes in the hillside, surrounded by sandbags and camouflage nets.

I was able to set up a small tent and do some dentistry, but at the time I felt distressed as I had impetigo on my left ear and upwards into my hair. The dental tent was on a slope, and as the monsoon was in full flow there was a permanent river running through it. One might say working conditions were difficult! A surgical team of two surgeons and an anaesthetist joined us temporarily and I was able to help with maxillo-facial injuries. There appeared to be Japs on all sides with our own shells passing overhead. We were on the outskirts of Kohima – lots of parachutes were hanging in the trees as most of the supplies came that way, or by mule and we were put on half rations.

Jap snipers were a problem. I was busy from 6 in the morning until dark, after which there was blackout. One day I went forward with the colonel to an Advanced Dressing Station (ADS) to see if help was needed with evacuation of casualties. We went down a steep bulldozed track in a jeep with chains. The mud was thick. Then we got into a Bren gun carrier but over the last mile we had to crawl along a bankside. The Japs saw us and fired, so we scrambled into the Chaung (river bed). They soon stopped as they were short of ammunition.

Having worked as the only DO in the brigade for several years, I knew most of the officers and many ORs very well. I had been to many of their parties, partly asked as a thank you, and so it was distressing to see them coming in wounded or hearing they had been killed – including three brigadiers. My impetigo had now been cured and I was able to shave and feel clean again, but I felt groggy as I had been given M&B[2]. We now heard of men being taken prisoner and tied to trees for bayonet practice.

Overlooking Kohima, we saw parachutes hanging on bare shattered trees, a nasty sight. Parachutes with supplies we had lost. I was now sleeping in my small dental tent on a stretcher across sandbags to keep me above the river rushing through the tent. Jap Zero aircraft were an irritation. Just an odd plane would appear as it did one day as I was talking to the padre of one of the battalions. He walked some yards away from me when a bomb dropped and killed him. We were all now told that the only way was forward, not that anybody had thought of retreating anyway!

I had a trench dug around my dental tent to see if that would help to keep the water out. I could do a little dentistry, but I was mostly dealing with casualties, and my batman was again able to wash my one change of green battle dress in a petrol can (top removed) of water, but of course it was never dry.

---

[2]   May and Baker 693. This was an early sulphapyridine bacteriostat and was very effective against a variety of infective organisms – *Editor*

Things were now quieter and I was asked to go back to Dimapore – forty-two miles away – and do some dentistry at Twenty-Two Casualty Clearing Station, so off I went with my batman. After a week I was glad to get back to the field ambulance. Dimapore was three thousand feet lower, was very hot, and I had prickly heat.

Joining the Fd Amb. again, I found then in a deserted village in bashas and they had been joined by the colonel of the India Field Ambulance who had been surrounded by Japs in Kohima and survived. He was awarded the Distinguished Service Order.

The rain was still torrential and now the dark brown leeches were around. They could even get through the lace holes of boots. Sitting up on end, they waved about and appeared to be looking around. A cigarette or match was used to get them off. One could not pull, otherwise it left a nasty place which went septic.

The Japs were retreating fast, and so we were given a rest period while the brigade regrouped. Of course, it was not a rest for me as now everybody needed a dentist, or so it seemed!

The slaughter of Japs had been high. They were starving and many committed suicide. We were now five thousand feet up and the malaria state was very high, although it was an offence not to take Mepacrine[3]. The other brigades were moving fast on to Imphal and we were two to three miles behind, so we could undress at night, and morning tea was not until 0630 hours.

As soon as Imphal was taken we moved further forward and settled down on a ridge eight thousand feet up. It was cool and pleasant, the river being in the valley, one thousand feet further down. We were told that we would have two to three weeks rest, but still had to send medical officers out to relieve sections. In the meantime, because of rainwater always getting into the dental tent, I was told that I could use a nearby bungalow. This was rather tank battered and I had to wait round a corner as there were some Japs in it. They were duly killed and we then had to get the bodies out and clean it out a bit.

I had to put up with a seventy-five millimetre gun firing in the garden, but this soon moved on. I had told the REME officers that using a dental foot engine was tiring and slow and as I was so very

---

[3] The first synthetic anti-malarial and forerunner of Paludrine. An unfortunate side effect was the production of a yellowish tinge to the recipient's skin – *Editor*

busy could they do anything for me? They fitted a six volt battery, dynamo, and a jeep headlamp on a stand and there was my electric engine and a good light. It created a lot of interest. General Grover came and had treatment, General Slim tried it, and Lord Wavell had a look.

I had to send diagrams to Delhi for the official War Diary, photographs were taken for GHQ and for the Assistant Director Medical Services, and an article I sent was printed in the *British Dental Journal*. I was now seeing fifty patients per day but insisted on having Sunday afternoon free. We were given more anti-cholera injections. Cooking could now be done with petrol pressure cookers – in the mud! Three Americans joined us here. They had volunteered to join the British before America came into the war, but could only join as medical aides and were used as stretcher bearer officers.

One of our medical officers went missing when out with mules to relieve a section. He turned up twenty-four hours later having apparently gone down the wrong path. He was ambushed by Japs, the mules stampeded, and he was lucky to get back. One of our men was killed with another stretcher party. Meanwhile I was busy trying to work out how to get my panniers on to mules, forty pounds each side, ready for the next move south.

In September 1944, things were quiet with patrols only over the Chindwin river. In October we were told that we could go on leave in turns. I was to be allowed fourteen days in the bright lights of Bombay, plus travel time. But that was to be in a week or two. Back in Kohima I went to look at the memorial set up there – we had all subscribed to it. It is, as you know, a large piece of quarried stone inscribed to the memory of the men of the Second Division:

> WHEN YOU GO HOME, TELL
> THEM OF US AND SAY,
> FOR THEIR TOMORROW WE
> GAVE OUR TODAY.

The stone was from a local quarry and was dragged up the hillside by Nagas. It was of just a rough shape and texture but was very moving. Lord Munster, Secretary of State of War, arrived and wanted to see my dental centre. We shook hands and he questioned me about the troops. General Montague Stopford also congratulated me on treating eight hundred and fifty men in the previous month.

After my leave I returned to Dimapore to find that three new RAMC stretcher bearer officers had joined us. The Fifth Field Ambulance dental officer had gone home and a new man had been appointed, but he was sent to join me for a week or two to get the hang of things before joining the Fifth Brigade. He was forty-one, which I thought was far too old for the job! The ADDS came to see us and asked me if I would like a more comfortable job in a hospital. I said, "No, thank you." We were on the move into jungle and were again sleeping in holes in the ground. By December 21st we had reached a point fifteen miles from Kalewa where the division hoped to cross the Chindwin river. And so we were told to celebrate Christmas.

A communion service was held in a Chaung at 0800 hours and I had a tarpaulin put up between trees with boxes and planks as seats ready for a party. At 1100 we went to Brigade HQ – a twenty minute walk – for a cocktail party. I was then asked to the Manchesters but refused, as I did not want to get tight before the men's dinner which we were to serve. I had had past experience of Manchesters' drinks. We gave our men twelve bottles of gin to share with three bottles of beer each. Before our dinner the brigadier and the brigade major, who was very drunk, came to see us and they spoke to all the men. We had our Christmas dinner at 1830 and had five guests from the Manchester Royal Scots and Norfolks, who all arrived very drunk. We were served with hors d'oeuvre, soup, a fish concoction made from tinned herrings, chicken, peas and potatoes, Christmas pudding and a savoury made with macaroni cheese and tomatoes, all from tins. Each of us had two bottles of whisky, two bottles of gin, and four bottles of sherry, but we had to share four bottles of brandy.

On Christmas Eve we were up all night and moved on so that we could cross the Chindwin at Kalewa at dawn. Manchesters along the track kept us in the right direction and protected us. And so on the 25th at dawn we crossed by a pontoon bridge. On the real Christmas Day we had bully beef, jam sandwiches, cheese and tea. We were now on half rations as there were parachute supply difficulties. A psychiatrist joined us. He saw some of the men with problems and some were sent back. My batman heard that his wife had had a baby. Obviously he was not the father. It took me some time to get him out of severe depression and to start to write to her again.

A message came that the recently-arrived dental officer who had joined the Fifth Fd Amb. – I mentioned him earlier – had been killed on Christmas Eve. I had always considered that it was a mistake sending him. A small Jap bomb from a plane had got him.

So many blokes wanted to see me for dental treatment that it was impossible to deal with them all. All our supplies were now coming by parachute, even parcels from home, the contents of which we shared. No bread now, only army biscuits.

Again I had some maxillo-facial work, a particularly nasty case this time that took two hours. The men fighting in the furthest away could be seen by us two to three hours after being wounded. One afternoon we were asked to go to a Catholic convent. Apparently the Japs had left it the day before and medical help was needed. I went with two medical officers and did the necessary as best we could for the nuns and priests. I was asked by a priest or nun (I don't remember which), "What can I give you?" I did not want anything but it was necessary to accept something and so I asked for one of the innumerable crucifixes on the walls. And here it is – I still prize it very much. The next morning a female arrived at my tent with a live chicken, also a gift. The people were always so generous. That chicken I regarded as a pet. It stayed with me until I left Burma, was named Matilda, laid an egg every day, and sat on my knee in the jeep when we moved.

On the move again in the Schwebo area. Here my best pal was wounded in the chest and flown back. I thought it would be the end for him, as we had found that chest wounds had the worst prognosis. He was the man (Lieutenant M. Freeman) who received the Military Cross at Kohima and survived. We were nearing Mandalay and were on guard a few hours each night in fox holes. I remember my batman always wanting to do guard duties with me and be at my side to protect me. I told him not to be so daft and to get some sleep. Later I heard that he asked the corporal, "Is the gaffer all right?" He was also good in that if I lost anything or had it pinched, a similar article turned up for me quickly with no questions asked!

By March 1945, I was the only dental officer in the division, one had been killed and not yet replaced, and one sent home. It was getting hotter: 100°F in the shade. For the next move I was given a four wheel drive truck and so was nicely comfortable with my batman, mess cook, and Matilda. Then Matilda disappeared. I was very sad, but she was found having made a nest with seven eggs in it.

It was now April 1945 and the DDMS (Brigade Corps HQ) had offered me a staff job with promotion in Ceylon (SEAC HQ). I was the longest serving officer in the Fourth Field Ambulance. For the first time I had to say that I had had enough of travel, heat and discomfort, blood and death. We were all tired of long distance travel on unmade road or bulldozed tracks, and days and days of army biscuits, and I had just heard on a radio how many people were at Brighton for Easter.

We had reached Myinyan and there was a dreadful smell on our site. We found five dead Burmese, each with their hands tied together. All five had been killed and pushed into a hollow by the Japs who had left the spot two days earlier – a terrible sight.

We were now told that the whole division was to be flown back to India. I read later that this decision was due to the fact that there were supply problems, but things were going well. Rangoon had to be reached before the monsoon started, and Mountbatten had plans for an attack on Rangoon from the sea. Also, Slim wanted the Seventeenth Indian Division to reoccupy Rangoon as they had been the troops beaten up by the Japs in the retreat to India.

My pet, Matilda, had to die. We boarded Dakotas and had a nasty flight to Chittagong. The pilot said that he had no time to get above the storm and so the trip was very cold and dark with rain and sleet rattling on the plane and violent ups and downs. We reached Chittagong after three hours.

Staying the night in Chittagong, I had a look round the bazaar. The next day we boarded a train and had an uncomfortable ride for eight hours to the Brahamaputra where the line ended. Here we boarded paddle steamers with comfortable cabins. Sailing in the late evening up the river, we arrived at a railhead on the opposite bank at 11.00 a.m. the next day. Then there was another eight hour train journey to Calcutta. This was an easy journey as there were lots of coolies to move baggage, berths on the train, and we had our own bedding rolls and stopped at stations for meals.

It was hot and sticky at Calcutta, but we had a good camp. I had arrived with one spare shirt and green slacks, and so now I could start to buy decent clothes ready for my move to Ceylon and a more comfortable life. After all those years with the division it was going to be a sad parting. However I was looking forward to seeing Ceylon and the Cocos Islands.

Of the three dental officers in the division, one had been killed, one was awarded a Military Cross, and I got promotion to a staff job.

HIMMLER'S SUICIDE
[With acknowledgements to
After The Battle (Volume 4)]

Heinrich Himmler was a close companion to Hitler after the Nazi party was formed in 1929. He became head of the SS, Hitler's élite bodyguard. By 1936 he had become Chief of the German Police. As Reichmaster of the Interior he commanded the RSHA (State Security), the GESTAPO (Political), KRIPO (Criminal), and SIPO (Barrack Security). Later he was responsible for the SS – Totenkopf-verbaende, the Death's Head concentration camp guard which operated the largest mass-murder system known to history. As Reichführer SS he expanded the military element of the SS – the Waffen SS – into an army of nine hundred thousand men. In addition to all these offices, he was made Commander-in-Chief Army Group Rhine from October 1944 and Army Group Vistula from January to March 1945.

On 30th April 1945, Hitler committed suicide and Admiral Doenitz, appointed in his place as Head of State, dismissed Himmler from all his offices. He was wanted by the Allies for war crimes committed on his orders.

Himmler went into hiding and adopted a new identity. On the 22nd May he and his escort were arrested, having presented forged ID documents on challenge. He confessed his true identity to his British captors next day, was placed under special guard, and his body searched. A medical officer suspected that Himmler might be concealing poison on his person and lastly, on examining his mouth, noticed a small blue phial sticking out from the lower sulcus of his left cheek. The MO hastened to clear out the object but Himmler, realising what was happening, clamped shut his jaws, swung his head away, crushed the glass capsule between his teeth and took a deep breath.

He died at 2314 hours. During the post-mortem Lieut-Colonel E. C. Browne, AD Corps, Assistant Director Dental Service, Second Army, was authorised, under secret cover, to take models of Himmler's teeth, write a dental chart, and report on dental condition. Major B. R. Attkins, AD Corps, assisted by supplying the materials and taking the models to the unit dental mechanic for casting and shaping. Only three masks were made and the original mould, face mask, chart and report are kept on display in the Royal Army Dental Corps Museum in Aldershot.

Post Mortem Examination To Establish Identification, Carried Out At 1100 Hours, 25th May 1945

The body was that of an adult male, well-nourished and physique up to average standard. Apparent age – middle forties. Post-mortem staining was present on points of pressure.

There was an oval scar, one inch by one and a half inches, on the upper border of the right patella. Small, slightly raised pigmental mole, two centimetres in diameter, in mid-line of back over seventh thoracic vertebra. Abrasions (recent) – two small circular abrasions over tendo achilles on both heels. Three small scratches on posterior aspect of left hand. Scratch four inches long passing vertically downwards over medial angle of left scapula.

General Description

Head: Average size, symmetrical, with a high, slightly receding forehead. Occiput flat with no marked line of demarcation at upper border of neck. Three furrows running upwards from inner angle of orbit.

Hair: Brown, generally thin; the hair receded from the forehead and there was a bald patch three by two and a quarter inches in occipital region. Very few grey hairs were apparent. The hair had been recently cut.

Eyebrows: Not heavy. On the inner third of both eyebrow the hair was growing in a vertical direction.

Eyes: Slightly protruding, colour – grey. Glasses. Right 5.75 sphere; left 6.0 sphere. Creases in skin under eyes not very pronounced.

Nose: Bones of bridge moderately high and well shaped, the nose increases in breadth acutely from the bridge to the anterior nares which were wide, the right being slightly larger than that of the left. The skin of the alar cartilages is drawn tight. The tip of the nose is slightly flattened and deviates towards the right. There is a faint cleft at the tip in the mid-line.

Face: Broad in joining the malar bones and narrowing towards the lower jaw. The cheeks are not full but there is a fullness in both parotid regions. The face is unsymmetrical, the left malar bone is higher than the right, the left cheek slightly fuller. Two pronounced creases run from the lateral tip of the nostrils on each side of the angle of the mouth. Mouth not large and no unusual features are apparent. The chin recedes in a marked manner and there is a cleft in the mid-line; the cleft is not very pronounced.

Ears: Average size, the right ear protrudes slightly more from the head than the left and the upper border of the pinns is somewhat bigger and broader. The fossae are deep in both ears and there is a fair growth of hair from the external auditory meatus. Immediately anterior to the tagus on both sides the skin of the face is creased in small folds which slightly overlap the anterior edge of the lobe of the ear.

Neck: Short and thick, marked fullness in submaxillary region, the line of the lower jaw is not well defined. Two well marked folds in the skin below the chin. Cricoid cartilage moderately prominent.

Chest: Well developed, normal shape, good growth of hair on anterior surface.

Abdomen: Normal fullness, not protuberant, pubic hair extending to umbilicus. No scars.

128

External Genitalia: Possessed no unusual features.

Anus: Two small tags of skin just external to external sphinctus.

Arms: Muscular , hands not large; fingers moderately long and tapering; nails cut closely at lateral edges with slight point.

Legs: Muscular and well developed. Feet normal in size and shape, no corns apparent or deformity of the toes.

(Signed) M. South (?) Capt. RAMC, Graded Pathologist, 74 Br. General Hospital.

Cadaver of
REICHMINISTER HEINRICH HIMMLER
REPORT ON DENTITION

[CADAVER examined at 11.00 hrs + 13.15 hrs on
25. May. 45 at 31.a. VELSENERSTRASSE,
LÜNEBERG.]

Signs and.
(Abbreviations employed are those authorized in
Regulations for the Medical Services of the Army,
1938, Appendix 13.)

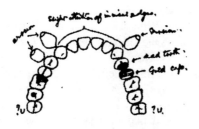

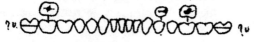

NOTES.

① Oral Hygiene – Good.
②. 8̅7̅ missing.
③ all fillings are of Silver amalgam.
④. Teeth well-formed.
⑤. Shade of teeth. (incisors, upper) – Shade 7. (Amersham Right)

25. May. 45.   Lieut-Col.
LÜNEBERG.   A.D.D.S. Second Army.
                  (Sd) G. R. ATTKINS. Major.
                      74 (Br) General Hospital.

SIEGE OF TOBRUK
APRIL 11th – DECEMBER
10th 1941

Within the fortress on 11th April were forty thousand troops, including seven thousand prisoners of war. Before the end of the month some twelve thousand were evacuated by sea. For the first three months the diet consisted of bully beef, biscuits, tea and vitamin tablets. The water ration was a gallon a day per man.

Captain Reuben Green, Army Dental Corps, arrived in Tobruk with Captain A. State during the siege. They embarked at Alexandria and sailed on the destroyer *Kipling*. In Tobruk harbour a lively reception was awaiting – bombing, shelling and pouring rain.

There were five AD Corps officers in the besieged garrison who at first were accommodated in the Italian Barracks high on the hill overlooking Tobruk. After dental surgery duties the dental officers assisted the medical teams by administering anaesthetics, dressing wounds and sorting casualties. Work greatly increased when the Eighth Army set out from Egypt to relieve Tobruk.

PRISONERS OF WAR – ARMY DENTAL CORPS PERSONNEL

Official records compiled after the cessation of hostilities (1939-1945) give the following bare facts concerning dental personnel who were made prisoners of war:

British Expeditionary Force – France and Belgium
Six Dental Officers – Eight Other Ranks.

Far East
· **Hong Kong**
Four Dental Officers – Four Clerk-Orderlies and two Mechanics.

· **Malaya – Singapore**
Sixteen Dental Officers – eighteen Clerk-Orderlies and twelve Mechanics. Three Officers and two Dental Clerk-Orderlies were reported missing, later presumed killed in action.

Middle East
Three Dental Officers and a number of soldier tradesmen of the AD Corps were taken prisoner by German parachutists in Crete when they invaded that country in 1942.

Germany
Captain Julius M. Green, a pre-war member of the TARO.

NB Some of the following stories reflect the spite and malevolence of the Japanese captors towards British and Allied captives. Despite the fact that the Germans had signed the Geneva

132

Convention, they too had committed atrocities and executed some Allied POWs captured after trying to escape. However, nothing can ever excuse the criminal behaviour of Japanese and Korean guards towards POWs in their charge.

THE ARMY DENTAL CORPS IN THAILAND 1942–45

[Colonel C. H. James, late Army Dental Corps]

After the fall of Singapore in February 1942 the mass of British and Australian POWs were concentrated in Changi, at the eastern end of Singapore.

Rations were very short, kitchen staff had much to learn about rice preparation and cooking, for there was nothing else. There were seven ounces of rice per day, and three to eight ounces of meat per week, so that a shred of meat might appear, but rarely, in one of the three light meals of rice issued daily. Furthermore it was difficult for grown men, used to a European diet, to accommodate the sudden introduction of this, an all-rice diet, which had been subjected to variable inexperienced cooking methods.

After a few weeks men became weak and debilitated, there was no spring in their step, and with much overcrowding, many succumbed to diarrhoea, dysentery, dengue and much failure in staying upright in the slouching conditions experienced. Later in the year, conditions in Thailand were worse due to the very lack of enough food to eat and the POWs already weak condition on arrival in Thailand from Singapore.

At Changi, several dental centres were set up, usually two or more dental officers to each centre. At Southern Area camp, one of three dental officers, three dental clerk orderlies and one dental mechanic, worked one outfit plus additional barber's chairs taken from the local village shop.

134

Two of our young AD Corps soldiers had a narrow escape from death in bayonetting of staff at the Singapore Alexandra Hospital.[4] They had been tied up, watching earlier batches taken out be bayonetted, but as their time came night fell. By morning news of capitulation had became general and they were released, to find their way to the POW compound at Changi and to join our unit.

Our supplies were greatly helped by an enterprising Malayan Volunteer Dental Surgeon who went back and burgled his own practice, generously sharing some of the proceeds with his dental colleagues. At these improvised dental centres, sick queues of a hundred men and more would form, but the gradual weakening with consequent reduced resistance to disease lowered the number of those attending as well as those operating.

At times, it was difficult to man the centre by more than one team, but the service never broke down completely, and we all took turns in visiting each other as we rotated in and out of hospital with our debilitating diseases.

Deficient diet after dysentery reduces one to permanent convalescence. However, the centre staff kept going and even produced upwards of a hundred dentures in its first six months. To watch Cpl Brandon, AD Corps, the dental mechanic working with a vulcaniser over an open wood fire was an education.

After a time, drafts of soldiers went to work in labour camps around Singapore (but the main body of POWs remained in Changi). Rumours spread that drafts of men would be required up north, with the added attraction that conditions would be much better with adequate food and running water. Around July 1942 the first draft left, some with MOs and DOs in company.

---

[4] This refers indirectly to a particularly vicious incident on 14th/15th February 1942 at the British Military Hospital, Alexandra Rd, when Japanese troops in their advance into Singapore, entered the hospital grounds and systematically went through all the wards and theatres, shooting and bayonetting patients and staff all the way up to the top floor. At or near the site (some staff were held captive to be killed later on) Capt. E. C. Cardwell, Capt. W. Walker, Pte S. M. Brooker and Pte L. F. Hayes, all AD Corps personnel, were murdered by the Japanese Army. An in-patient of the hospital, Capt. J. G. Brown, AD Corps, was also murdered.

For DOs, difficult problems arose over unserviceable quantities of equipment. Too much might have to be discarded en route, but too little, all too early, might prove quite inadequate. By September 1942, so many had left that a medical team of twenty officers, including our padre and one DO and staff, was duly alerted. Our turn came in November when we entrained in steel covered rail wagons.

By privilege, one truck was allocated for MOs, some twenty-three men, the normal quota being thirty. This permitted some to sit, with crouching for those unable to sit for lack of space. We were also privileged to have the sliding door open.

These trains were known as square-wheelers. No adequate time at stops was given for proper relief. Buckets of food were handed in at certain points up the line. For the sick it was grain (and the constipation was unusually ghastly). The step height of the train was too much for most to get in and out.

After nearly four days we arrived at Ban Pony, some thousand miles north of Singapore. As our camp was not ready, there we remained for a time. The station and environment was littered with the disregarded accoutrements left by previous parties, who had marched straight off up the jungle (to build their own camps of an evening and work from then during the day).

As there was a shortage of guards, our party was for a time given a comparative measure of freedom (walking up the street and visiting other camps, hearing news, and fearing the worst).

The food was an improvement on Singapore. There were canteen facilities supplied by vendors and at them we were introduced to the Thailand duck, that laid eggs in such a profusion, priced at three cents each, and to whom every prisoner, however alien, owes a great debt. Bananas and peanut cake were also obtainable. These canteen items stood us in good stead except for times when the Japanese, for no apparent reason, refused to allow them.

Our comparative freedom lasted for two weeks until one night by the light of the moon. During the small hours a faint hum was heard overhead, followed half an hour later by faint crumps as Bangkok was bombed. This gratifying interlude happened on two or three nights at the height of the moon each month.

Loose POWs were quickly rounded up and the remnant of this hospital party found themselves in Nong Pladuk, three kilometres down line, a base supply camp for the railway. A good selection of

MOs and DO service was already being given at this camp, with some fine work. Two years later this camp was heavily bombed with many casualties in February 1943, the remnant of this hospital party was moved sixty kilometres north-west to a small market town at the foot of the jungle – Kanchanaburi.

The working party at this camp was fairly fit, but the first draft of men arriving from up country camps was a shock and they soon started to fill the partially constructed camp.

They journeyed by open truck on jungle track, or by barge without escort, sometimes travelling seventy kilometres in forty-eight hours. At worst, as many as twenty-five percent might be dead on arrival (but usually only one or two bodies out of seventeen to twenty men would be lifted out dead). A man of six feet might weigh six stone. Starvation, dysentery and malaria were rife, but when cholera struck later, they died on site and were incinerated.

Eventually the camp filled up to Japanese standards of sixteen to an open atap hut, each man had three feet of bamboo slat fence bed, to reach a total distribution of one and a half thousand in camp.

Our understanding of the term 'fitness' underwent some change. A man fit to work was one who could stand up, though perhaps with a little help!

A short term hospital case would be in care for six months. An ill man had little hope, but might be prone or sitting for two years (and even then occasionally he might improve).

It might appear that there was not much to do for a DO in such sorry company. But there was plenty (there was a small open room, with a shutter for setting up a field chair and panniers).

Routine dentistry was practised as near as possible to normal. Sterilisation took place in a mess tin over a charcoal burner. Local anaesthetic – Planocaine – looted by a rating from a naval base and handed in to the dental centre; a large carton of out-of-date tablets crushed up as required with a brown inky substance, proving better then nothing.

A large bottle of cocaine snow was obtained from a Changi chemist store made up to a 0.5% by our RAMC dispensers, as required. This was used with discretion, but a local anaesthetic was avoided as much as possible, owing to infection risks, and cocaine was also dangerous.

Extractions were instructively performed in cold steel, for a man in bad pain suffers only relief after extraction.

Cavities were black type, interstitial filled with silver and all simple cavities with Zn-0 lining and cement filling. Minor oral operations were performed only when essential.

Pte John Moody, AD Corps, the dental technician, did sterling work not only in nurturing our slender stocks, servicing equipment with great care, but also even carrying on as DO when the in-camp dentist was down with diptheria, detailed instructions sometimes being given from his sick bed. A testament to this service was the good running condition of nearly all the equipment, especially when a move in 1944 allowed no means of transport and it had to be left to a dental surgeon then serving as a gunner.

Our great advantage was the value of having a worthwhile job to do in times of stress, boredom and dismay.

Twice, the dental outfit, complete with personnel, was confiscated by the Nips but a spirit of lack of co-operation, and a lack of understanding on the Nip side, led to a reunion to our own. Some dreadful deals, unworthy of a professional man, were undertaken – for example, to supply Victoria Metal Crowns in exchange for cash for genuine gold rings.

Generally speaking, dental treatment of the Japanese hosts was carried out normally but without endearment to encourage return visits. For instance, when a Japanese was waiting, the POW in the chair was encouraged to shout loudly from time to time to give the impression that much was being done. Thus a very useful impression was created.

Gingivitis was rare, but boulders in the rice caused many broken cusps. Case output was lessened, due no doubt to lack of sticky carbohydrates.

The dental staff participated in many extra curricular activities, such as burial parties, wood fuel parties pinching sleepers from the railway, and bamboo cutting parties. Sometimes massed burial parties had to attend to the sad pressgang camps full of Malays, Indians and Chinese who had no knowledge of kitchen, latrine and camp maintenance procedures. These unfortunates would die in their tracks by the dozen. There were also pig rounding up parties, when the Nippon pigs mysteriously escaped on a warm spring evening.

In these parties the DO and his camp staff were fitter than the men detailed to work and it became necessary to encourage the guard to visit the local 'Saki' shop or 'brothel', so that work arrangements could be adjusted for those who could not walk very well.

One young MO said that two years before, under the strictest supervision and as a newly qualified man, he had six patients in his care at his teaching hospital of some six hundred and fifty beds. He now had three hundred and fifty patients all desperately ill, most unable to do more than sit up. He had no medicine and he doubted if he could ever tell the story to his consultant and expect it to be believed.

There was no news. The *Nippon Times*, published in English, spoke of the allied troops retreating in North Africa in a western direction and how a Japanese aviator out of ammo shot down his American attacker with a rice rissole, and in another air battle despatched one by a sword cut!

The operators of a 'canary' (radio set) in the adjacent camp were tortured to death, so extreme care therefore had to be exercised.

Visits from other DOs and their patients frequently brought something newsworthy and authentic, but care had to be used in dispensing the good word for fear of a tracing back to our own illicit source. Very rarely a mail bag would arrive, but the chances of anything for those in any one camp were not great.

At most, camps contained some factor of occupational therapy. In ours a cigarette rolling factory was managed by the DO. The Nips didn't like this, and one very unfit man was struck by a guard for not going out to work, resulting in his death and the Nip's consequent trial at a War Crimes Tribunal.

In 1943, the state of the prisoners was disquieting. Death at the current rate would have left no one alive by 1945. But with completion of the railway, the workers came down the line in 1944. Thereafter parties only returned to make good damage done by frequent RAF raids.

The evening Arrow-Head flights were so characteristic that one evening an orderly flight of twenty-seven were hardly noticed to be flying, without hearing the beating of wings. They were at long last RAF, and from then on some spectacular displays of attacks on adjacent camps were seen, including that on the famous bridge.

We saw the largest number of planes on 6th June 1944, a significant date – all destined for Bangkok – but as the allies advanced so the POWs were moved further eastwards. We had to leave our equipment and took skeleton packs only to Makom Nyok, ninety kilometres north-east of Bangkok. The damage to the railways and to the city greatly delighted us.

In our most remote camp, there was no opportunity for exchange of news. But in July 1945 some guards committed hara-kiri quite openly. Later there were rumours of an atom bomb, which although disbelieved continued to circulate.

Finally we were released as an Allied Officer and team walked into camp and set up a radio station.

So the graves that had been dug in the fortress for ourselves were not used for their intended purpose.

Flags of all nations represented suddenly appeared from sewn up doubled blankets, and were flown aloft.

Supplies were dropped in, and cattle driven in on the hoof. But we had no ideas on how to manage the new drug called Penicillin!

THE
BANGKOK-MOULMEIN
RAILWAY

Shortly after the surrender of Singapore on February 15th, 1942, all European POWs were concentrated in the Changi Military area of Singapore island, which was divided into divisional areas. Dental officers were sent to all areas and carried out fairly normal dental treatment.

In June 1942, I was sent as Dental Officer to a party of one thousand nine hundred men which proceeded to Thailand as an advance party for the building of the Bangkok–Moulmein Railway. We were sent to Banpong on the Singapore–Bangkok Railway, some fifty miles west of Bangkok.

Nearby were one thousand two hundred other POWs from Singapore with Captain E. Martin as their Dental Officer. I brought with me a set of forceps, elevators, six hand instruments (excavators, plastics and scalers) ten ounces of Novutox, and a small supply of zinc oxide and oil of cloves and one or two other drugs. Cavities were prepared using a chisel and excavator, and filled with zinc oxide and oil of cloves.

After four months in Banpong, we proceeded to Chungkai, about forty miles north and some three miles from the small town of Kanchanaburi. Shortly after we arrived there in October 1942, thousands of POWs from Singapore arrived to start building the railway, and with them was Captain E. Smith, AD Corps, who came to my camp. The camp strength was then five thousand with another three thousand five hundred men at a subsidiary camp two miles further north, this total of eight thousand five hundred men comprising Number Two POW Group. Other POWs further south, comprised Number One POW Group, and thousands further north were included in Number Four POW Group. I had by this time almost exhausted my small supply of anaesthetic and drugs and I had not received any from the Japanese, despite many requests and the fact that I was expected to treat them if necessary.

Captain Smith had similar equipment to mine but his supplies were untouched, as he had just come from Singapore. I received permission from the Japanese to go to Kanchanaburi to purchase drugs with our own money (i.e. money subscribed by the officers from their pay). At a chemist's shop in Kanchanaburi I was fortunately able to buy six grams of Planocaine powder, which we made up into a one percent solution and some oil of cloves, which enabled me to carry on.

I had a dental chair constructed of bamboo and string, which was designed and made by Capt. Spaulding, Indian Artillery, after the pattern of the field dental chair. I worked in a bamboo and attap hut, the drawing of which is copied herein. Captain Smith went further north with working parties in January 1943, leaving me in Chungkai.

I was able to make contact with Capt. C. H. James Army Dental Corps, who was in a base hospital at Kanchanaburi. Captain James had adequate dental equipment with him including a dental engine and a portable vulcaniser. I was able, with the permission of the Japanese, to take several patients about twice a month to Kanchanaburi Base Hospital, to prepare cavities with the aid of Capt. James's foot engine.

This wasn't of great use considering the thousands of men who were in the camp, but it enabled me to maintain valuable contact with Capt. James and his equipment. I was able to replace various instruments such as mirror heads and drugs, both for myself and for Capt. Smith up country, from Capt. James who was very helpful. I was able to send some of our home-made local anaesthetic and oil of cloves to Capt. Smith, with whom I was in contact frequently.

Chungkai became the biggest Base Hospital camp in Thailand, as thousands of sick men, worn out by starvation, disease and overwork poured into the camp, until it had a strength of over ten thousand by the middle of 1943. Drugs were very scarce indeed, but I obtained a supply of one percent Novocaine from the Japanese, which was quite good and we made up a two percent solution of Percaine which had been sent in with other drugs by the Swiss Consul in Bangkok. Zinc oxide and oil of cloves continued to be the main standby for restorations.

142

In September 1943, I managed to order and obtain a fair amount of dental cement and some Bayers Novocaine from underground sources in Bangkok. This I shared with Captains Smith and James. I was also able to get some dentures repaired through the same source, but this took so long to arrange that I had to find other methods of repairing dentures. One method was to drill holes on either side of the break with a broken probe, and lace up the denture with floss silk, and when this ran out, with silver wire.

Another method was to rivet pieces of aluminium from Dutch mess tins over the broken denture. I was able to have a full upper and lower denture made for a RAMC quartermaster, and a full upper denture for a medical officer, by Captain James who had a small amount of rubber and a vulcaniser.

An excellent mechanic, Pte Moody, AD Corps, also a captive, acted as his orderly. When I ran out of wax for the bite stage, more was obtained from old candles.

The rubber plunger of my syringe having perished, I was able to have fresh washers made of the uppers of old boots and fitted to the syringe which proved satisfactory. I had a syringe of Capt. James's repaired by this method, which he was still using eighteen months later.

In March 1944, Capt. Smith came back to Chungkai with the rest of Group Two, and we worked together again. By this time, Capt. James had moved away from Kanchanaburi, but I was able to contact an Australian Dental Officer, Captain S. Simpson AIF at Tamarkan Camp about three miles away.

He had good equipment, including a foot engine, and I was able to replenish my supplies of needles and also to give him some anaesthetic of which he was very short.

In June 1944, the first big supplies of Red Cross drugs from the outside world arrived. In this was a large quantity of Novutox, some zinc oxide and eugenol. Our worries about local anaesthetic were now at an end. In fact we still had a fair amount left when the war ended fifteen months later.

Among our patients were several cases of fractured jaws caused by beatings up by Japanese soldiers. I treated one soldier and Capt. Smith treated two officers with fractured mandibles. I believe other dental officers had similar cases.

In January 1945 Tamarkan Camp was closed. It was situated close to an important railway bridge, which was bombed frequently by Allied planes, and the camp itself was hit and twenty POWs killed.

Captain Simpson thus joined Smith and myself in Chungkai. In February 1945 all officers except medical and dental officers and padres were taken away, concentrated in Kanchanaburi, leaving us with the men. We carried on until June 1945, when Chungkai Camp was closed and we moved to Tammuan Camp about twelve miles south. I had to leave behind my bamboo dental chair which I had used continually for two years. After less than two months at Tammuan, the war ended.

The work I did was mainly extractions and temporary fillings with a fair amount of gum treatment. The diet in my opinion did not have much effect on the incidence of dental caries among the prisoners. Much of the dental deterioration was due to the lack of toothbrushes among the men, and the stagnation areas brought about by failure to remove food from the gingiva and interproximal spaces. I saw many cases of avitaminosis manifested by a sore tongue and angular stomatitis. Vincent's disease was rare, considering the crowded conditions in which we lived.

By Captain D. Arkush, a wartime Army Dental Corps dental surgeon posted to the Far East and captured by the Japanese. This is his story, when as a prisoner of war sent to the notorious Death Railway in Siam (Thailand) in 1942.

DENTAL POW IN THE FAR EAST 1942-45

On the capitulation of Singapore in February 1942, all POWs were moved out to Changi. These included British and Australian and numbered several thousands.

It was at once apparent that the Japanese were not going to obtain and provide medical, including dental supplies, so from the start we had to resort to improvisations of every kind in order to attempt to afford any kind of dental treatment at all.

Within the first fourteen days of our incarceration, Brigadier Lucas of Malaya Command had to be taken to Tanglin Barracks by Japanese staff car. Captain Finlayson, AD Corps, requested permission to accompany him as it was thought that there still might be some dental supplies in the Tanglin Dental Centre. As a result of this trip small supplies of amalgam and filling materials, also local anaesthetic, were made available. These were a useful addition to the field dental supplies which odd units had brought into Changi with them.

The first dental surgery (as such) was set up on a first floor verandah space in Roberts Barracks and immediately types of improvisation commenced. The spittoon, which was the enamelled iron field equipment type, was a source of trouble as it required frequent emptying. The 'Sappers' who were interned invented a 'fountain' type spittoon for us which was mounted alongside the portable dental chair. This incorporated a running water scheme which did not require emptying. With these primitive facilities the small number of dental officers in this area were able to afford emergency dental treatment and, while supplies lasted, routine dental treatment in some instances, but this did not last for more than a month or so.

Working parties were already in operation in Singapore and were partly housed in River Valley Road POW Camp. Word was received through an interpreter that several cases of severe toothache had arisen and the Japanese would not allow these men to travel to Changi for treatment. It was therefore decided to send Captain W. F. Finlayson with a corporal and parts of a field dental outfit to this camp, if the Japanese would agree.

After considerable haggling this was agreed. Conditions in River Valley Road Camp were most unpleasant – overcrowding was such that three men had to live in a space of six feet by three feet. The atap huts were alive with bugs, etc. and skin conditions were rampant. Dysentery too was on the increase, and great difficulty in sending serious cases back to Changi was experienced.

The dental officer commenced his treatment of the acute cases on the site of a mud drain, out of which had been scooped a seat with mud back support. Twenty-eight cases were dealt with on his first day and efforts were made by the OC of the camp to find a small space where he could set up the portable chair and carry out further treatment. This was important as it was already rumoured that the POWs there were earmarked to go up country where absolutely no dental facilities existed.

Again, improvisations were made. An ingenious operating light with an old highly polished tin can as reflector was constructed by a grateful patient as the inside of the huts were very dark.

It is worthwhile mentioning that small surpluses of dental materials were occasionally brought into this camp by members of working parties who had managed to contact Chinese residents, while out on working jobs. Contact with Changi was very difficult and was only possible if our interpreter Major Wilde (later Brigadier) managed to get out and back in a Japanese truck. Incidents, of course, were frequent and the Japanese method of punishing the camp was to turn off the water for two days, with disastrous consequences to acute dysentery cases.

While here, the dental officer was transported complete with field outfit to Japanese Headquarters where he was directed to treat senior Japanese officers. This had one good side to it as one of the officers treated brought some dental supplies to the camp. We assumed that

146

he must have found a Chinese dental supply shop functioning in Singapore.

From a clinical point of view, deficiency diseases were becoming prevalent and the oral manifestation of these were often seen. It was impressed on the POWs that the maintenance of good oral hygiene was paramount to prevent these oral conditions going septic, but by this time, the supply of toothbrushes was practically finished and improvised ones were made.

By the end of June 1942, the POWs in River Valley Road were starting to go up country and the dental officer and orderly were called back to Changi by Lieut Colonel T. Pearson, the Assistant Director of Dental Service (ADDS) Malaya Command.

In Changi, movements were afoot. The Senior Officers (Colonels and above) were being got ready to go to Japan. Working parties were being assembled into large groups called 'forces' to go north to Siam for the ghastly experience of building the Burma-Siam railway. The POW Hospital as such was becoming a combined British and AIF Outfit under the command of Colonel Craven and had hundreds of cases including the battle casualties, vitamin deficiency, and so on.

The survival of these sick patients was becoming an acute problem as the Japanese stopped a man's pay if he went sick and also cut his rations. As a result, hospital staff gave most of their so-called pay to try and purchase extras for the patients. Chinese contractors were being contacted by working parties and were gradually becoming accepted by the Japanese. Great caution had to be exerted, as any suspicion of messages being passed brought terrible retribution by the Japanese.

As food was priority number one, there was little chance of trying to get material and dental supplies through these contractors, and in any case, all the Rolex watches and Parker pens which were negotiable for Japanese currency had mostly gone. Colonel Julian Taylor, who asked to remain with his patients and not to go to Japan, was doing good surgical work with his colleagues and carried on this magnificent effort right through until the release in 1945.

Colonel David Middleton looked after the anaesthesia and advised on the treatment of maxillo-facial casualties. He also gave the dental officers some very fine lectures which where appreciated. He too carried on right through until his release from Kranji (Woodlands Camp) POW Hospital in 1945.

Dental treatment was not confined to the hospital area alone. Mr Callum, a civilian dental practitioner in Singapore and a POW as SSVF, managed to salvage some of his equipment and did a magnificent job in what was called Southern Area. The AIF too had dental officers working in their areas, but as the numbers in Changi diminished these dental officers went with 'Forces' up country. When Selarang Barracks were evacuated, the POW Hospital moved there.

In 1943 when the Japanese decided to put the remaining POWs in Changi Jail, they decided to move the POW Hospital out to a site adjacent to the Naval Base at Kranji (Woodland Camp). This was a hutted camp surrounded by rubber trees and on the main road to the Johore Causeway. The camp had been occupied by Indian troops and they had left behind many cats which they evidently looked upon as sacred. The protein value of these was too much for the incoming POWs and there was not a cat to be seen in a week!

Captain W. F. Finlayson, AD Corps, was the dental officer selected to go with the POW Hospital staff. The hospital camp was commanded by Lieut Colonel J. C. Collins, RAMC and the staff were a mixture of AIF and RAMC personnel. Colonel Julian Taylor was in charge of the surgical side (British), and Major Graves the medical side (British), Lieut Colonel Osbourne, RAAMC surgical side (Australian), Lieut Colonel Cotter-Harvey, RAAMC medical side (Australian).

A portion of the end of a hut was allocated for a dental department where a field dental chair and part of an outfit was set up.

By this time, a few patients were beginning to arrive from up country and they were in an appalling condition. Efforts to produce vulcanite-type dentures had previously been made over in Changi but the problem of vulcanising the mixture of raw latex from rubber trees with laterite dust and fibres of wood had been unsuccessful.

Here in Kranji, we had ample latex supplies so the problem was tackled again. After many failures we finally produced a partial denture after sixteen hours vulcanising with home-made charcoal as the fuel. During our stay in Kranji over one hundred dentures were produced and several somewhat toothless POWs were available to chew their meagre rations. Oral manifestations of Beri-beri, Pellagra, Aribo flavinosis continued to be seen, but the setting up of a purveyor of rice polishings, which were thrown away by the Japs and contained the eleurone layer with vitamin content, greatly reduced these conditions.

By themselves, rice polishings are most unappetising, but by various ingenious methods the cooks managed to incorporate their sawdust-like material into more attractive and appetising forms. At this time too we were able to obtain limited supplies of red palm oil which was used in cooking.

Semi-permanent conservations, using oil of cloves and zinc oxide as a base were experimented with and certainly stopped further caries spreading until proper conservations could be inserted.

The reader has to remember that the dental officer had only a few hours a day to do professional work as even hospital staff had to form working parties outside the camp each afternoon. This was sometimes heavy manual digging and cultivating gardens, which, when productive, the Japanese wired off and took over for themselves. Other working parties, especially in 1945, went by truck up into Johore where officially teak trees had to be cut as supports for 'rice stores', but as we ultimately found out, they were to be battle positions to resist air attacks.

By mid-1944, our rice ration was down to half a teacupful per day and we just managed to survive with odd extras obtained through Chinese contractors. As time wore on, the situation became more and more precarious.

Occasional gifts of dental supplies were brought into camp by Japanese officers and ORs who had been treated. With experimentation and improvisation, dental treatment was afforded whenever possible. The old lesions of the oral mucosa were not often seen in the latter stages as many of the affected patients had died and probably the intake of rice polishings kept them in abeyance.

Such conditions as a perforating ulcer probably from an extensive Vincent's infection in a very debilitated patient were rarely seen. This case actually occurred in Changi in 1943. Also seen at this time were several cases showing oral manifestations of scurvy (vitamin C deficiency). The classical petichial haemorrhages, loosening of teeth and hyperaemea gingivitus, were often observed.

Aribo flavinosis revealed itself chiefly as a painful chielosis and angular stomatitis while the 'raw beefy tongue' of pellagra usually accompanied the three Ds (dementia, dermatitis and diarrhoea). Local applications did little to ameliorate these painful conditions, and in any case, apart from some carefully saved chromic acid, there was nothing to apply.

When we finally did receive the odd Red Cross parcel there was very little of dietetic value in them as we did not get a regular supply.

We were finally released in August 1945, and having seen all our hospital cases off by air and sea, our staff were evacuated by air and sea to the UK.

The undermentioned were AD Corps prisoners of war working with Captain Finlayson:

Corporal Firth Private Gilbert	Dental clerk-orderlies
Lance-Corporal Latter Private Brennen	Dental mechanics

THE POW SPECIAL – SIAM-BURMA

[H. Brennan, LDS., RFPS, Dental Surgeon, Kilbirnie, Ayrshire, a wartime commissioned dental surgeon captured by the Japanese]

Figure 12 is fairly self explanatory. The crude chair from a log, with bamboo armrests, webbing was the back support, and the sole luxury was the head rest – a piece of sorbo rubber stolen from the seat of a Japanese truck.

Despite its apparent crudity, the 'chair' was quite functional and a multiplicity of operations were carried out in it. Zinc oxide was in fair supply – begged, borrowed, and stolen from various sources – and oil of cloves was distilled by a POW chemist (we could get the raw cloves on the black market) in a Heath Robinson apparatus. The Japanese medical sergeant, Fukunda, bought me supplies of cloves out of his own money when he went on leave to Bangkok – one of the few good Japs I met.

At his instigation, a wooden chair with movable back and headrest, on rachets (old barber's chair principle) was made for me by the camp carpenters in about June or July 1943 and this was an improvement on my original.

The new 'mod-cons' included a charcoal brazier on which we could boil up instruments.

A SORT OF DENTISTRY –
ON THE RIVER KWAI
[Basil Peacock, MC TD, LDS RCS]

During a full and versatile life I have practised dentistry in some queer places, but the queerest was up the River Kwai years ago.

I was serving as an Artillery Officer in Malaya when a Japanese shell knocked me out. On coming to, I found myself a prisoner of war. Some months later I was in the jungle of Thailand building a railway and bridging the River Kwai along with several thousand other Japanese slaves, the most inadequate tools, and on a diet of rice plus a morsel of protein when available.

After nearly three years, when the railway was completed, forty per cent of the prisoners were dead and the remainder in poor shape. We were returned to a base camp at Kanchanaburi to await our next task.

Though there were one or two officers of the Army Dental Corps amongst the prisoners, there was none at the camp, but oddly enough there *was* another combatant officer, a pilot in the RAAF, who was a dentist in civil life. When I revealed that I was one of the profession, we decided to team up.

My status as a prisoner went up; it could not have been lower with our captors. As a 'ha isha' tooth doctor, I was taken off labouring work for more skilled duties. The Japanese were quite anxious personally for some sort of dentistry, as they had no means of obtaining treatment for themselves and toothache comes to the unjust as well as the just.

Like most Eastern races, they were tooth-conscious and their numerous gold crowns were always coming adrift. Personally I had no objection. After three years as a ganger and labourer, any job was better than digging huge trenches round the camp, which the more pessimistic, with good reason, thought to be our mass graves.

Our surgery was set up in the so-called hospital hut, where the desperately sick lay closely packed on bamboo slats, touching each other. It was similar to all the other huts; bamboo posts supporting palm leaf roof and walls. We cut out a piece of roof and propped it up to gain light to work.

The equipment consisted of a chair of bamboo poles lashed together with split bark, a foot engine, one very loose handpiece, a metal syringe with only one needle, one pair of lower root forceps, and three upper forceps. These must have come from Singapore with part of a field ambulance kit. The lower root forceps caused endless trouble to us and great distress to the patients as there was no pivot pin. We used nails and bits of wire as substitutes but all broke under pressure.

There were some medical tweezers and a chisel and we made small instruments. The engine was minus a cord; a real problem, as string or rope was unobtainable. The usual fastenings of the East – rotan or bark – were unsuitable. The problem was solved when a water buffalo was slaughtered for food. A strip of hide was cut, pared down and softened. It worked reasonably well. Half a kerosene tin made a steriliser when placed over a charcoal brazier. We had to prepare the charcoal by roasting wood in a primitive way.

In fact, we had to begin in the primitive way for everything, much like the old painters making their own paints and doctors their own medicines from simple ingredients. Fortunately there was a small amount of zinc oxide and an ingenious Dutch chemist made us some oil of cloves from the flower buds by double distilling, using a still made from kerosene tins. He also made us some crude alcohol by distilling a potent batch of rice wine we used to brew in secret from rice water, palm sugar and banana skins when the 'Nips' were careless. A nearby kapok tree provided a substitute for cotton wool.

As a form of occupational therapy we set some of the lighter sick to work, filing down coins and articles of silver to make the basis of amalgam, hoping we could find some mercury.

Our establishment was completed by the appointment of a dental attendant, a captain in the Malay Volunteers and a particular chum whom I was anxious to see released from working parties. I think I told the Japanese he was needed as 'holding down man" and as their own medical dressers carried out such duty they thought it reasonable. He contributed a large crystal of copper sulphate which he had been carrying about for years.

His duties included making appointments. These were written on the concave side of a split bamboo, which has a parchment-like surface. His main duty was to provide charcoal and fire for the steriliser. This was no simple task, as at that time matches were non-existent. Before the clinic opened he would make fire with flint and steel, plus a piece of kapok in a bamboo tube. If this method failed, he would visit the cookhouse several hundred yards away and rush back with a flaming branch, rather like a messenger with a fiery cross and light a coconut oil lamp made from a tin and a wick of cloth.

Our worst headache was supplied by the sole hypodermic needle. Fortunately it was the old-fashioned type with a blob of lead at the butt end. The Dutch engineer repaired the butt frequently, using a primitive blowpipe and lead coin.

There was no cement or local anaesthetic and we had to depend on a procession of Japanese patients to obtain supplies in this way. A 'Nip' soldier would appear, making uncouth noises with a shell crown in his hand or with a finger in his mouth to indicate that he required dental care. We would be interested and sympathetic but would shake our heads sadly, saying, "No cemento. No sleepo medicine (anaesthetic). Nippon soldier go to Bangkok and buy medicine, okay, we do!"

He would depart and return several days later with quite a selection of useful material picked up in one of the thousand Chinese drug stores in Bangkok, all of which have the most weird collection of goods which are usually many years old. The 'Nip' would hold up the packets asking if they were Japanese, American English, or another make, and invariably he would select the English brand for use on himself.

We always acted ethically and gave the Japanese as kindly treatment as our own patients, which was considerably kinder than they received from their own doctors. We used all the remaining materials for the prisoners and when the next 'Nip' appeared we shook our heads again and repeated the performance.

The dental department provided another useful service in concealing valuables, especially precious metal. At this time the Japs had begun intensive searches and stripped us of any trifles of value, pens, pencils or even letters and paper. My colleague, a most nimble-witted officer, persuaded the camp commandant that silver was useful for making shell crowns and repairing teeth, so we were allowed to retain some.

Thereafter we acted as a safe deposit for articles that other prisoners had managed to conceal. Some were kept on show as a shop window, the remainder in ingenious hiding places in the surgery. Often a Japanese patient was sitting on a silver mine.

Cigarette cases were particularly useful for splints. Fractured jaws were not an uncommon consequence of beatings by guards. One interesting case was treated in the following way. As soon as our railway was completed, the Allies set about destroying it from the air. This was heartening, as by it we could judge that we were winning. Unhappily, because most camps were close to the bridges and lines we sustained casualties.

After one raid by the Americans we had eighty casualties. During the RAF raid which destroyed the main bridge over the River Kwai, a large lump of turf and bamboo fell on the head of a British officer crouching in a trench. His chin came down heavily on his knees and his mandible fractured in two places.

It was essential that a prisoner should be able to eat everything of his meagre diet, which was little above starvation level, so inter-maxillary wiring was out, even if we could find some wire. We decided to make a cap splint. My colleague did most of the practical work, assisted by various experts in improvisation. Trays were made from bits of kerosene tins and an impression was taken with candle grease. This was cast with cement from the railway. A sand mould was prepared, and a die and counter-die poured with a mixture of lead and coins.

A Dutch officer produced the lead, which, I surmise, came from bullets. The necessary heat was produced from charcoal and rough bellows of buffalo hide. A segment of a silver cigarette case was swaged and the splint fixed over the patient's teeth with cement, left over from the treatment of a Japanese. The patient was wearing the splint in reasonable comfort when we were released.

A few weeks before the end of the war I was sent with a party to a distant camp. After a most arduous and wretched journey, we finished with a march of forty-eight kilometres in eight hours in a temperature of ninety-six degrees Fahrenheit. Some stores had been sent by lorry but every article of medical equipment was impounded by the Japanese.

Fortunately for us, a horrible sentry, known to us as The Undertaker, developed a foul apical abcess and came to us for treatment. When he at last understood that I was helpless without tools, he arranged that together we would steal them from the store hut. We removed all the medical supplies that we could collect. Sitting him down on a fallen tree in a secluded spot, I performed a grisly but successful operation. Pathetically, The Undertaker was executed by the Allies some weeks later for brutality and murder of prisoners.

A fortnight later, a British officer developed such a septic mouth that the only available doctor and I decided to clear his teeth to save him from general toxemia which might be fatal. The doctor had half an ounce of chloroform, the last of any form of anaesthetic. We laid the patient down on the ground and before he could recover, as he was only semi-unconscious, I could hear shouting and someone caught my arm. I shook off the hand, swearing at the delay. Finishing the extraction as the patient became violent, I turned and said, "Who was that clot shouting during an anaesthetic case?"

"Ich," said a Dutch Marine. "I come to say the war it is finished."

We bent over the bleeding patient and shook him till he understood. "War finishee. Alla sodjers go home."

ON LOOKING BACK –
HONG KONG
[Captain George Johnstone, AD Corps]

To write about day-to-day experiences in a prisoner of war camp
should be a simple task, but I find, in retrospect, that the period of
some thirteen hundred and fifty days behind Japanese barbed wire
was so full of incident that it becomes a problem to know what to
write about to give a proper impression of that life.

There is so very much which cannot be told and so much more
which to the outsider might seem commonplace and childish. I think
I may be forgiven if I assume that a full appreciation of the
circumstances of that life is denied to him who has not experienced it.
How can the uninitiated know the thrill of writing from memory the
full works and music of one of the Gilbert and Sullivan operas, or of
recalling the lines of some classic in the realm of literature, or of
making from empty cigarette packets and other scrap, the necessary
properties and paper money for that excellent time-passing game
Monopoly?

Or can they understand how, even at a time when morale was at
its highest and life seemed to have relatively few snags, there was
always that undercurrent of doubt as to whether our captors would
appreciate our latest attempts to amuse ourselves or whether they
would read into our humble efforts all sorts of insults to themselves?
Or how can anyone know the real joy of receiving a Red Cross food
parcel without having lived on a diet of boiled rice and filthy green
vegetables or stewed chrysanthemum leaves?

But life did not consist simply of varied emotional experiences.
There was plenty of work to be done, and in fact, without some work
to do, one might soon have become mentally deranged. Perhaps the
outstanding thing about work was the variety of tasks with which one

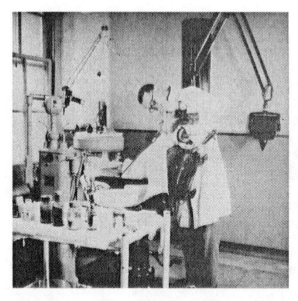

*Fig. 16   Forbes Finlayson as a dental specialist working in
the UK. (top)*

*Fig. 17   Forbes Finlayson visiting FARELF as Corps Director in
1967 (Pte. A. Muldoon RADC, in the middle, was murdered
by the IRA when serving as a Sgt. in N. Ireland). (bottom)*

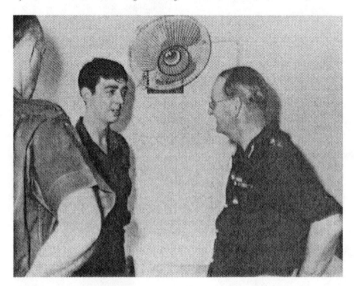

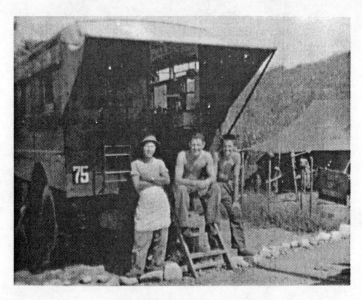

Fig. 18   A mobile dental team on active service in Korea. (top)

Fig. 19   A tented waiting room, active in Korea. (bottom)

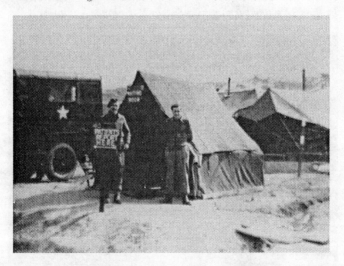

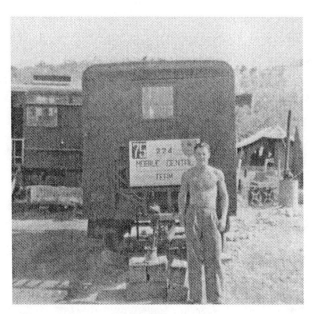

Fig. 20   A mobile at rest for a period in Korea. (top)

*Fig. 21   'Hearts and Minds'. Headman and children await surgery
time, Long Pasia, Borneo, 1964. (bottom)*

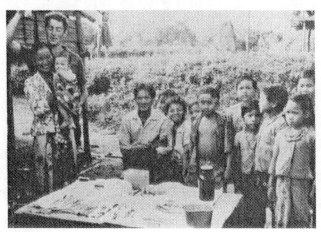

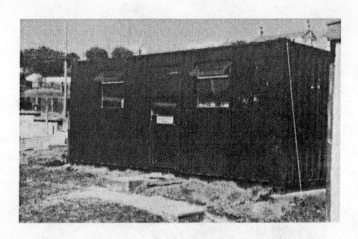

Fig. 22   Containerised dental unit, Falklands War. (top)

*Fig. 23   Mobile dental caravan replacement being transferred from
site besides Military Hospital, Stanley, destroyed by
fire. (bottom)*

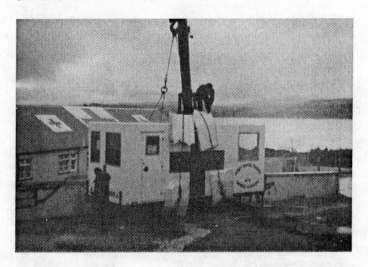

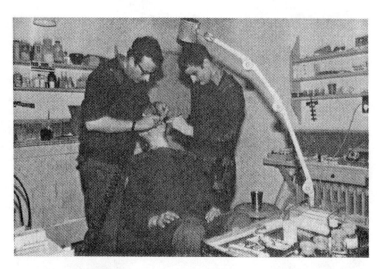

Fig. 24   Dental staff at work on temporary shift, sharing laboratory, at Stanley. (top)

Fig. 25   The Gulf War - mobile dental teams, dental care staff at Al Jubail. (bottom)

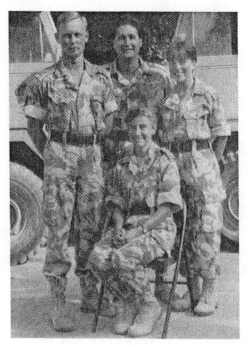

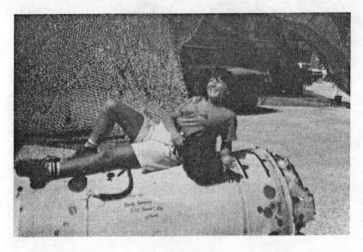

Fig. 26   *Major Kate Fisher relaxes aboard a dud SCUD. (top)*

Fig. 27   *Tuhen, Saudi Arabia 1990 - Major B. Nuttall visits a US Marine Corps dental unit. (bottom)*

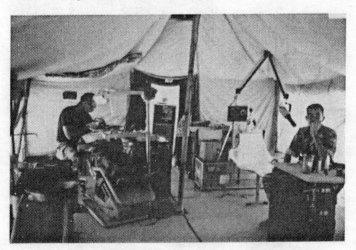

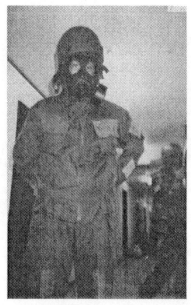

Fig. 28   Capt. Mark Earl in full NBC kit expecting the worst, most of the time. (top)

Fig. 29   Gulf staff of 205 General Hospital Capt. P. Grainger and Pte. S. A. Taylor RADC. (bottom)

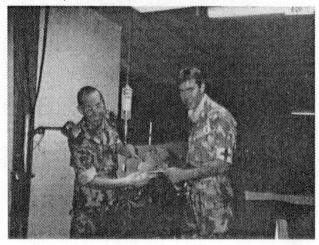

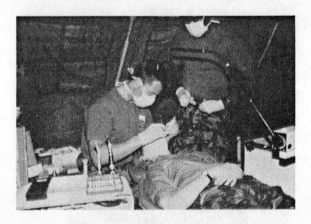

Fig. 30   Dental team at Bugoguo working under cover of a factory as the camp was frequently under artillery fire. (top)

Fig. 31   Sector West Medical Platoon Operation Hanwood Centre: Capt. G. Janos RADC as OC. (bottom)

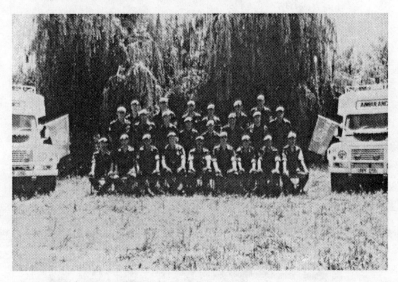

could occupy one's time. We were fortunate in that we were not forced to work for our hosts and all that we did was for ourselves. It was a rather wonderful example of a communal system of living. Sharing was the rule both in work and in leisure.

One could choose between gardening, wood chopping, vegetable cleaning, sanitary duties, boot repairing, haircutting, tailoring and repairs, the camp workshop, the poultry farm or giving assistance in the camp hospital. This latter duty was most remarkably and capably carried out by volunteers who had no previous experiences of or training in sick nursing and there are many who will ever be grateful to them for their gentle care of the sick.

It is rather amusing to look back on some of the more outstanding contrasts between the normal peacetime occupations and those brought about by necessity; the banker-nursing orderly, the policeman-patcher of shirts and shorts, the stockbroker-baker, the lawyer-boot repairer, or the shipping magnate-bricklayer.

Everyone found something with which to occupy his time, either for the benefit of all or in his leisure hours, to increase his own knowledge.

Classes of all kinds were conducted, mostly in the open air – book-keeping and accountancy, motor mechanics, languages (about fifteen in all), elementary classes for medical students, history, literature, architecture, and many others. Some of the classes were in the nature of general lectures and perhaps ought to be thought of more as entertainment. In this field there was great variety, band concerts, musical shows, plays, camp farces, and so on. It would be difficult to know who had more pleasure from this aspect of camp life, the players in rehearsals and performances or their audiences; but certainly all were, for a time, transported from the sordid circumstances in which we lived to some better and more pleasant place.

I have purposely refrained so far from mention of the worst side of our life, the bad and inadequate food, bad general living conditions, lack of medical facilities and drugs, because that is the part that everyone wants to forget. It was a hard time, with little in the way of respite from trying conditions. We were ever conscious of the trigger itchy guard, when the slightest misdemeanour, true or alleged, was productive of a slapped face, if one was lucky, or a beating with a bamboo pole or sword scabbard if one was rather less

158

fortunate. All that is over and done with, and perhaps it should be left without saying more.

What about our reaction to the freedom which came with the end of the war in August 1945? Perhaps the following description of a simple but dignified ceremony of 'Raising the Flag' will help towards an appreciation of what it meant to us to have reached the end of a long period of deprivation, want and disease.

All ranks paraded at a few minutes before eight o'clock on Saturday morning after the news of the Japanese surrender had leaked through to us. The band played a rousing march as we assembled. There we stood in varied garb, some wearing much patched shirts and shorts, others in uniform rather obviously rescued from the bottom of a kitbag, but for us this was something of an occasion and all were determined to put on a good show despite sartorial deficiencies. Faces and frames were thin but there was a new light in our eyes and we had a certain pride of bearing, for were we not now free men?

A short service was held terminating in the order, "Attention," and to the strains of the National Anthem, the Union Jack was slowly hoisted. Some there were who tried nobly to sing what had been for so long in the category of forbidden music but for most of us the occasion was charged with so much emotion, that we were content to enjoy the band's gallant effort.

A simple ceremony, but one full of symbolism and hope. What thoughts were in our minds in those short moments? What of our comrades who were not with us on that day – those who died in battle or as prisoners, those in hospital too weak and ill to come on parade? Suddenly we were aware that our return to normal life and home and loved ones would not be all joy and gladness, that there would be gaps in the former circles of friends, and our thoughts rested for a moment on the many sacrifices which had been made to gain deliverance for us and peace for the world.

Later, with a fuller knowledge of all that had been happening in the world outside the barbed wire, we realised how we who have endured and were not overcome must all strive to banish for ever the guilty madness of war.

With Captain Johnstone in captivity were the following Army Dental Corps personnel:

Lieut. Col. J. McCurdy – ADDS China Command
Capt. N. L. Fraser

Capt. D. E. Wallis
S/Sgt. G. P. Shorthouse
Sgt. A. W. Smith
Sgt. G. F. Taylor (drowned on transfer to Japan)
Pte. D. Pratt
Pte. R. W. Bairstow (died in Japan after rescue from the *Asamu Maru* [torpedoed])

COLDITZ – EXTRAMURAL ACTIVITIES OF A DENTAL OFFICER POW

Captain Julius M. Green, a pre-war member of the Territorial Army Reserve of Officers (TARO) until it embodied in 1939, decided to write his story for his family and his children. He does not call it a history, but an account of the experiences of one man and his interpretation of events in which he took part.

Captain J. M. Green was the Dental Officer of 152 (Highland) Field Ambulance when taken prisoner of war at St Valery-en-Caux. His first prison camp was at Tittmoning. In January 1941 he was informed that he was to be moved to another camp in North Germany. The senior officer took Captain Green to the bedside of a young officer who taught him how to use a code for sending messages in his letters home. The War Office intercepted this mail, decoded it, before sending it on to the recipient.

Captain Green's next camp was Marlag and Milag Nord at Sandbostal. Here he was able to treat the prisoners, glean information and send messages without detection. His patients were mainly Royal Navy and Merchant nationalities. It was at this camp that he came across a sub lieutenant RN who defected to the Germans and betrayed his compatriots. Later Captain Green appeared as a witness for the prosecution when the sub lieutenant was tried and convicted of high treason in 1946.

Prisoners taken at the St Nazaire raid were confined in a separate compound. Captain Green devised a system for signalling to the commandos and sent them congratulations from London.

His involvement with the commandos was discovered after an escape attempt and he was transferred to camp E3 Blechammer. Here he persuaded three company sergeant majors to send allotment forms purporting to allocate twenty-five pounds to their wives. Afterwards, the forms had been treated to contain sketches and maps. Weeks later the disgruntled trio had letters from their wives thanking them for the money! The messages had got through the German censors.

Late in 1943 Captain Green was transferred to Oflag BF at Marisch in Czechoslovakia. In January 1944 he was sent to Oflag IVC Colditz. The sub lieut. was brought into the camp and Capt. Green was assigned to watch and keep him clear of escape attempts. Later he admitted to being a traitor. Some mention of this is made in the book *Colditz - The German Story* by Hauptman Eggers, the German security officer at Colditz.

Throughout his captivity Captain Green used his powers of observation to good purpose, and as a result sent home information of interest and value by using his coded messages.

The time came when Green sensed that he needed a change of clothing – his service dress uniform had been lost when his truck blow up at St Valery and altogether he was feeling rather scruffy. So to boost morale and to restore his confidence in his dealings with his German captors he set about getting something new. He persuaded a seaman (also a prisoner), who had been a tailor before the war, to measure him with a piece of string, which was in turn measured off against a ruler. These measurements, together with a cheque written on a piece of plain paper, were sent to his tailor in Glasgow and about two months later a 'service dress' complete with buttons and badges arrived, and fitted perfectly (now kept in the Corps Museum).

Records of Work done whilst a POW are now lost, except for that from February 1942, when he left Milag Westertimke and went to Stalag Eighty-eight (E3) at Blechammer, up to the late Autumn 1943 (exact date unknown).

Fillings 1,500; scalings, etc., about 150; extractions, 2,350; dentures, between 470 and 500. Plus temporary crowns, denture repairs, surgical extractions, and acting as anaesthetist for the MOs in various camps. Attendances for treatment – at least 4,700.

Dentures were made from Paladon and the teeth from Palafont in plaster moulds taken from a few sets of porcelain teeth. A limited supply of local anaesthetic and filling materials was obtained from the German Red Cress. The instruments were mainly from the Germans, plus what he managed to salvage from a field kit.

Most of the prosthetic materials were obtained from the Dental Depot in Bleiwitz with canteen funds, helped out with Red Cross cigarettes and silk stockings obtained from the French workers' black market, in exchange for Red Cross cigarettes and chocolate. Some were improvised from tin cans, builders' plaster and candle grease.

In Marlag and Milag he worked from December 1940 to February 1942 – six days a week sometimes, but generally five days per week. There were up to six thousand seamen of every nationality, and ninety-nine percent had not had dental treatment for years, and many never. While in Milag he was also in charge of camp hygiene and was the anaesthetist in the camp hospital.

He was moved from Milag after doing two weeks in solitary, having been suspected (correctly) of being implicated in an escape attempt by the chaps from St Nazaire and sent to E3.

At Colditz he was not allowed to practise and was held as a security prisoner, classified as *'Deutsch Feindlich'* (hostile to Germans).

THE LONG MARCHES – A PRISONER OF WAR

[Colonel K. C. Blanthorne, MBE]

Early in the morning of the 12th June 1940, personnel of 153 Field Ambulance RAMC made their way through the lush Normandy countryside towards the Channel coast. Our hope was that the Royal Navy would carry out a repetition of Dunkirk and evacuate the Highland Division from the beaches of St Valery-en-Caux. The previous night a RN destroyer had successfully embarked the divisional wounded from this small Franch port.

However, our luck was out and the enemy advance was too swift. Held down in a wood some miles from the coast by fire from the tanks of Rommel's Armoured Division, we, along with Scottish and French infantries, with whom we had become inextricably mixed, were forced to surrender.

A long and painful march into Germany followed and the start of nearly five years as a prisoner of war, firstly in an officers' camp in Bavaria and then in soldiers' camps in Poland and East Prussia. After only a few weeks in Oflag VIICH in Bavaria, I was transferred to Stalag XXA in Poland where, with RAMC officers, we provided medical and dental treatment for the thousands of British, French, Polish and Belgian prisoners of war in the area.

My work was carried out with instruments and materials provided by our captors, but as the war progressed and we were in touch with home, equipment was received from Britain and from the International Red Cross in Switzerland. During this time Corporal Jim Kettle, AD Corps, assisted me in the surgery and other willing workers from the infantry were quickly trained to assist.

After the fall of Crete in 1941, Australia and New Zealand medical officers and a dental officer joined us as prisoners, so at least some help was available to share the dental work. My colleague, Captain C. C. Cook, NZDC, and I were able to provide more conservative treatment for our patients than had been possible previously.

When the German attack on Russia began, thousands of emaciated Russian prisoners were brought into new camps in our vicinity but we were allowed no normal contact with them. Typhus raged amongst the Russian prisoners, and many of our medical officers, at great risk to themselves, worked daily amongst the Russians to give them medical attention. Conditions in the Russian camps were terrible and a great number of men died from typhus, starvation, and indiscriminate shooting by their guards.

For a time we had in one of our camps in Stalag XXXA a number of army and RAF officers, including that indefatigable escaper, Group Captain Douglas Bader. A visit to the dentist was looked upon as a chance to make an escape and this happened a number of times, two officers escaping through my surgery window while a diversion was staged in the waiting-room to attract the attention of the guards.

After some two years in Thorn, I was transferred to Stalag XXB at Marienburg in East Prussia, working on a mixed bag of Allied POWs from the camps and farms in the area. Here I was aided by my good friend Corporal 'Taffy' Rosser, AD Corps, whose cheerful personality did much to alleviate the tedium and depression from which we all suffered from time to time after long years behind barbed wire.

In this camp, with reasonable equipment and materials, we were able to provide dentures for some of the Allied soldiers who had had to struggle on for so long in an edentulous state. The new acrylic resin Paladon, supplied by the Germans, was used for the first time by us and proved to be remarkably successful.

We seemed far from the war but our secret radio kept us informed of its progress. We were convinced of ultimate victory for the Allies but doubted at times whether we would be too old and decrepit to enjoy our freedom when it finally arrived. However, release came dramatically and unexpectedly for us.

SECOND ARMY SITUATION REPORT BY SIGNAL

Second Army Dental Sitrep No 1. 21 Jun (D+15)   SA/99/5/Med

21 Jun 44

D.D.D.S.
21 Army Group

1. A.D.D.S. landed on 18 Jun 44 at 0.20 hrs (D+12).

2. Dental arrangements appear satisfactory.

3. Minor complaints of fracturing of dentures in masticating biscuits.

4. No 212 M.D.U. landed on D + 13 and reported to Second Army HQ at 11.30 hrs on 19 Jun 44. Was directed to HQ Army troops, and has opened for treatment of local tps. on site 50 yds from HQ (Med).

5. No information has yet been received at 1 or 30 Corps HQ regarding arrival of remaining M.D.Us - A.D.M.S. Army Troops is investigating delay.

Ext 924,
Rear HQ
Second Army
IN THE FIELD.
ECB/DEI.

(Signed) E.C. Browne, Lt.Col.
for D.D.M.S.
SECOND ARMY.

Copy to: Brig A/Q.
War Diary (2)

A strong Russian attack along the whole of the Eastern Front against the German armies began in early January 1945. Towards the end of that month, increased tension amongst our guards and the civilian population in the streets outside our camp became apparent.

Suddenly evacuation of the civilian population of the town was ordered and German tanks took up position in the streets and in the surrounding countryside. Our guards became very concerned about their probable fate if captured by the attacking Russians and appealed to us to demand that we be removed to the west. However, we were determined to stay and in any case we had no wish to move our seriously ill patients in the chaos of a major retreat and the cold of an East European winter.

When the Russian advance reached the outskirts of Marienburg and shellfire increased, we removed our sick and ourselves to the two cellars in the building and to the trenches we had already prepared in the grounds. For two days, the Germans and Russians fought around us. We admitted to our camp hospital both German and Russian wounded, and we suffered a number of casualties amongst both patients and staff.

Eventually the firing died down as the Germans retreated across the river. Early in the morning of the third day of the attack, a cautious glance through a window overlooking the street outside showed a Russian patrol in white camouflage uniform moving with care up the road towards us. With the aid of a wounded Russian officer, but keeping our heads well down, we made known to them who we were. Soon we were suffering bearhugs from the Russian soldiers, many already celebrating their capture of the town and in an alcoholic haze were following a successful search for liquor.

For about two weeks we awaited fulfilment of Russian promises to transport us to Moscow while resisting all attempts to get us to volunteer to join them on their march to Berlin. In this period we melted snow for water and lived off the cows the Russians brought in for us to slaughter, and from what was to be found in the abandoned houses in the nearby streets. We were objects of much interest to the Russians and were visited constantly by Russian officers and by hard-drinking trigger-happy soldiers.

The fact that the Germans were shelling the town daily was an added spur to our constant request for evacuation and eventually primitive horse-drawn carts were produced, our sick loaded on to them and away we marched through the Russian lines of communication, going east.

On our way back through the devastated villages with large numbers of German dead around, the Russians arranged food and shelter for us at night, but after about ten days these arrangements collapsed. After we had moved our sick to a Russian field hospital we found ourselves virtually on our own. Soon we divided into small groups as we scrounged lifts on Russian trucks, but with little knowledge of where to make for.

We lived off the land, sometimes fed by Polish families, sometimes by the Russians, as we made our way east, deeper into Poland, joining the ever-increasing number of Russian and East European civilians released from German labour camps and on their long trek home. Also on the road were long columns of German prisoners of war on their way to Russia and imprisonment. Many of these dropped out of the line of march suffering from wounds and exhaustion. They were instantly despatched by a bullet in the head.

Once, we were befriended by a young Pole who took seven of us to his home, where we shared food and accommodation for some days with a tough Russian tank crew and two pretty Polish girls and their mother. Our presence was welcomed by the Polish family and eventually the girls accompanied us into Warsaw, where they were able to join relatives.

The city of Warsaw was a heap of rubble after the Polish uprising against the Germans there. Terrible reprisals were taken by the Germans against the Polish Secret Army when the insurrection failed, but life went on in the suburbs of the city. Here we were looked after by many kind and patriotic Poles, anxious to show their gratitude to the British. They advised us to make for the town of Lubin in the south-east of Poland, where rumour had it that a camp had been organised for British and United States POWs by the American Legation in Moscow.

More lifts in trucks, and eventually we arrived in Lubin. We were much relieved to find that our Polish friends' stories were true. An American colonel from the Legation was demanding and getting some help from the Russian Town Commandant, and despite the Russian bureaucratic obstruction, a train of cattle trucks and some rations was organised, and we set off on the long, slow journey through snowbound Ukraine to Odessa on the Black Sea coast.

After some days in Odessa we heard the unbelievable news that the Cunarder Samaria had arrived to take us home. When we embarked we could hardly believe our luck that once more we were free.

RUDOLF HESS

An early incumbent of Number 720 Army Dental Centre Berlin, Captain Andrew R. Nunn RADC, wrote evocatively of his experiences in Berlin during his posting starting in the summer of 1959. This is not quite a war story, but this one episode highlights an important hangover from World War Two:

I had not been many weeks in Berlin when I had a telephone call from the prison at Spandau, which at the time held Baldur von Schirach and Albert Speer in addition to Rudolf Hess. The request was for a dentist to come immediately as Prisoner Number Seven had toothache.

Cancelling my appointments for the rest of the morning, I left for Spandau. Having identified myself at the guard room, I was escorted through a series of huge gates, up some steps, and finally into the inner sanctum. My guide now left me in the hands of the inner guard. We were in a large hall, straight ahead was a barred gate leading into a cell block. To my left was a smallish room with two high windows. It was barely furnished as a medical treatment room with an examination couch, a drug and instrument cupboard and a writing desk. In the middle of the room was a metal, folding chair and foot operated treadle drill, standard field dental equipment.

I was familiarising myself with all this when my patient entered. He was dressed in an ill-fitting brown corduroy suit with the figure seven prominent on knee and elbow and on his back. He wore no belt, no tie, and his shoes had no laces. I recognised him immediately. It must have been those thick bushy eyebrows which were so familiar to anyone who had grown up in Britain during the war years. My patient was Rudolf Hess.

Walter Rudolf Hess was born 26 April 1894. He was Hitler's deputy leader of the Nazi party, a cabinet member, and head of the Nazi Party Organisation. He joined the fledgling Nazi party in 1920

and quickly became Hitler's friend and confidant. His flight to
Scotland in 1941 caused a sensation at the time. He had been in
various prisons, including the Tower of London, ever since. Later,
he was to commit suicide in Spandau in August 1987 at the age of
ninety-three.

When I met him, he would have been sixty-six. He presented
with an acute infection of the lower right first premolar. The tooth
was part of fixed bridge replacing 4/5. My problem was not in
removing the tooth – it was so mobile I could have done that with my
fingers – but of cutting through the bridge. It was made of some
strange metal with which I was unfamiliar, certainly not gold. I
remember thinking it strange that such a man, formerly a powerful
Nazi leader, would have such cheap-looking dental work in his
mouth. I asked Hess when the bridge had been made. With a shrug
he said, "In another life."

I tried, to no avail, to cut through the bridge using the treadle
drill. I was eventually able to loosen the crown on the first molar and
remove the bridge and tooth together. I separated the crown at my
own dental centre and returned to the prison that afternoon to re-
cement the crown on 4/6.

What were my impressions of Hess? Was he insane, as was
supposed? Was he an impostor as put forward by the former RAMC
surgeon, Hugh Thomas? I have no specialised knowledge as to his
sanity. We spoke, but mainly about his dental condition. I do recall
that there had recently been an air crash with consequent heavy loss
of life. Hess, who had access to newspapers, made some comment
about it. We had a short conversation agreeing what a tragedy it was.
He seemed a rational human being to me.

It was many years after I wrote this that I read *Hess: A Tale of
Two Murders* by Hugh Thomas. In this book, Thomas puts out the
theory that the man in Spandau was not Rudolf Hess. Hugh Thomas
is a surgeon who served out a short service commission in the
RAMC. He gained a lot of experience in gunshot wounds while
serving in Northern Ireland prior to his posting to Berlin. He was
interested to read in Hess' medical records that he had received two
GSWs in the chest during the first world war and was keen to see
how the wounds and scar tissue had resolved in the intervening forty
years.

He became suspicious about the man's identity when, on
examination, he could find no scar tissue. Further research

convinced Thomas that the aircraft in which Hess took off from Munich on 10th May 1941 was not the same one that crashed in Scotland. If Major Hugh Thomas' theories are true, Hess was murdered by the Nazis and it was an impostor who crashed in Scotland and was to spend the remainder of his life in prison.

Do I have anything to add to this mystery? Perhaps, if I could see Hess' pre-war dental records! Some information was released in 1992 and I have a cutting from *The Daily Telegraph* dated 7th June 1992 from which I quote:

> Dr Thomas interviewed Kathe Heasermann, the assistant to Hess's pre-war dentist, before her death. She claimed that Hess had no bridgework in his mouth... If Wednesday's revelations show there was bridgework in the mouth, the man who parachuted into Scotland in 1941 and was found guilty of war crimes at Nuremberg was not Hess, said Dr Thomas...

On reading this article I wrote letters to *The Daily Telegraph* and to the man who wrote the article, telling what I knew. I had no reply to either letter, neither have I been able to find what 'Wednesday's revelations' were. It may not solve the mystery but I can vouch that the man in Spandau did, very definitely, have bridgework.

It remains a mystery.

MY PART OF THE MALAYAN EMERGENCY

[Captain E. J. Bowen, RADC]

My captaincy had come through and I was granted leave to get married. While on my honeymoon I had a telegram ordering me to report with full kit for service in the Far East. Three weeks later I was on board a troopship as Dental Officer of the Sixteenth Field Ambulance.

We embarked at Southampton wearing battledress with the new RADC blue and red shoulder titles. These with the new cap badge and service dress buttons I had got while on my Officers Basic Training Course in Aldershot in January 1948. In my uniform case I had an issue of olive green tropical dress. I did not realise how terrible I looked in it until we got to Singapore and saw personnel in their local tailor-mades.

It took four weeks by trooper to reach Singapore. *HMT Dunera* was the last of a small fleet taking out the Second Guards Brigade to deal with the Malayan emergency that had been declared on 1st May. The unit to which I posted was the Brigade Field Ambulance. Under Brigadier Erskine, who was lost in an Auster over the jungle later, we were to clear up the mess in six months. It lasted in fact ten years.

Shipboard life was most enjoyable after rationed England. Trips ashore at Port Said, Aden and Colombo were memorable occasions for a young man away from England for the first time. The sight of a dhow under full sail, the swarms of fishermen standing in their canoes off the coast of Ceylon, flying fish and the sight of Achin Head Sumatra are indelible memories.

Having treated some of the ship's officers, I got in on a ship staff net and the social life was hectic. I was quite glad to reach Singapore.

Coming down the gangway with a sore head, I was accosted by a middle-aged man wearing sandals with a crumpled white shirt and shorts. Brusquely acknowledging that my name was Bowen, I learned that this was Colonel W. L. Pearson, Deputy Director Dental Service (DDDS), Far East Land Forces. An immediate change of attitude on my part.

After a fortnight under canvas in Nee Soon I travelled up country by road convoy to join the advanced party of my unit at Sungei Besi near Kuala Lumpur. Here I lived for three years with the Third Battalion Grenadier Guards. Living with them under canvas, I could afford a bottle of mineral water a day and still meet my mess bill. It was at Sungei Besi that I made the worst joke of my life. Having aroused some interest by saying I had served with the Guards during the war, I went on to say I had been in the Home Guard. No one spoke to me for a long time.

I first set up my panniers in a tent but later moved into a wooden hut, built on piles and with a thatched roof, in Sixty-four Reception Camp in Kuala Lumpur. I had said to my CO that it would be best for the dental officer to be located at a central point in the brigade area where men could come in for treatment in transport collecting rations. That the point I chose was the capital of Malaya was fortuitous. Colonel Clarke must have approved of my reasoning because he moved the whole unit in later.

For one year I used my field kit with good effect. Then, as the emergency showed no signs of ending in six months, Colonel N. F. Smith, by then DDDS FARELF, posted me to a static centre in Kuala Lumpur and I could at last get my wife out to join me. I handed over to Major 'Jumbo' Strange, who got a mention in despatches during his tour of duty with the field ambulance.

My unit, Number 911 Army Dental Centre, was in the HQ Malaya District cantonment. I had a wooden building at first with a thatched roof, which was later replaced by asbestos sheeting. I fell foul of the Assistant Director Medical Services, Colonel (later Major General) P. F. Palmer by trying to carry on a sick parade during the transition. I restored my position unwittingly by creating a garden outside the centre. Only later did I discover that an interest in gardening was a passport to his approval. An interesting feature of the garden was a tree sacred to the Hindus who laid flowers and burned lamps at its foot.

My two years at KL were uneventful despite the emergency. Travelling was restricted. Outside the cantonment we had to carry arms. Going to a night club wearing a white sharkskin dinner jacket and a holstered pistol made an odd combination.

I took over from Lt Col B. J. Swyer, the last ADDS of Malaya District and also OIC Number 911. He was a man of meticulous accounting accuracy. During my appointment Number 911 ADC also moved into my building, when we gave up part of the civil hospital on the building of BMH Kinrara. With Captain Wilf Jackson and his successor Major S. J. Gittings there was no friction despite our cramped conditions. With Lt Col G. E. Nettleship life was rather hectic. He carried stores accounting to an extreme. Once he was very angry to be a towel deficient. To my horror I found I was one in surplus. I threw it through a window in his part of the building as if it had been red hot. I was quite glad to leave Malaya, which I did in September 1951.

Captain E. J. Bowen went to Malaya in 1948 after a term in London as dental surgeon to the Olympic Games competitors. He eventually became the Director Army Dental Service as Major-General and was awarded the CB.

KOREA – UNDER THE 38TH PARALLEL
[Official Report by Major W S Y Mackie, RADC]

In August 1950, Twenty-nine Infantry Brigade Group was mobilised to proceed to Korea, to form part of the United Nations Forces there.

The dental cover for this force was Numbers 223 and 224 Mobile Dental Teams CMDTS) and additionally the dental section of Twenty-Six Field Ambulance, together with the Specialist Dental Officer of the Number Twenty-nine British General Hospital.

The two mobiles and field ambulance section each had laboratories – the first time, I believe, that a dental technician was on the establishment of a field ambulance.

The officers of these units were all regular serving officers and the other ranks were all reservists. Some of these reservists had to be replaced for compassionate and medical reasons.

Number Twenty-Six Field Ambulance, and Numbers 223 and 224 MDTS were all formed at the Army School of Health, Mytchett, and two months were spent assembling equipment, stores, vehicles and kit. As part of the stores to be taken to Korea, a special six months reserve of medical equipment was authorised.

The two mobile teams came under command of the OC Twenty-Six Field Ambulance, who was also the Senior Medical Officer of the force.

During this formation period there were parades and inspections prior to embarkation. All personnel had their embarkation leave, and by the beginning of October all units were ready to move.

The three dental units which formed the dental cover for the brigade travelled in three ships.

The Twenty-Six Field Ambulance, on the *Empire Pride*; Number 223 MDT on the *Empress of Australia* and Number 224 MDT on the *Empire Fowey*.

This was arranged so that routine treatment which had been started for the reservists in the UK, the main percentage of the force, could be continued throughout the voyage which lasted from thirty-five to forty-two days, depending on the ship. The amount of work to be done was quite considerable and the time available for routine work short.

On the *Empire Fowey*, Number 224 MDT was allocated one bay of the isolation hospital on A deck for a dental centre. The equipment used was a field kit, which was part of the ships stores.

On route, medical supplies and x-ray facilities were obtained at each port of call.

On arrival at Pusan, all three units proceeded to Suwon by rail. Rear parties of drivers were left at the transit camp to await arrival of vehicles. The stores of 224 MDT were aboard the *Empire Fowey* and these stores were taken to Suwon with the unit. The driver remained at Pusan to bring the vehicle.

During the time at Suwon the stores were unpacked and repacked to reduce space and a tentative layout for the surgery and laboratory was planned. After two weeks the unit stores and vehicles had arrived and the whole brigade moved north to take up its place in the line. This move involved convoys for long trips which took about two to three days to reach Pyong-Yang.

The majority of moves were done in convoy, with either the Coy HQ or the HQ of Twenty-Six Field Ambulance. Where this was not the case, the move was either with another unit or the move was independent. Long convoy journeys were at times unpleasant, due in the summer to dust and in the winter cold winds. In the main the roads were poor and only in and around Seoul were there tarmac roads.

In winter, snow and frozen ground made the job of windproofing tents and the penthouses difficult, but the use of sandbags removed the trouble and made the taking down much easier, besides making them more windproof.

In the initial stages of the campaign, a limited number of buildings were used and they made life much easier, but latterly the use of buildings was discarded and tentage was then the main question. The American Army supplied quite a large number of square tents which were of an ideal size and could be erected by six or eight men. As time went by, supplies of tentage became available and more problems were solved.

In the spring of 1951 the OIC Number 223 MDT obtained an office truck. This was converted by the workshops into a combined surgery and laboratory. The two side tents were used as sleeping and storage accommodation. This gave an enclosed surgery and laboratory, which was ideal. This vehicle was taken to Japan when 223 MDT was sent there for work at J RHU. This set-up was first class with one proviso – if any mishaps should occur, no replacement would have been available.

The main idea of the mobile should be to keep canvas to a minimum and of such a type that it only required the staff of the unit to erect without help. Another form of surgery was used by the DO of the Indian Field Ambulance. A 160lb tent was used as a surgery. This had to be dug out inside to give ample head room, but again one end had to be left open and this was not so good in the winter.

Prior to the formation of Number One British Commonwealth Division, the evacuation of patients after Tweny-Six Field Ambulance was through the American chain to Pusan, there to Twenty-nine British General Hospital.

In the American chain, at anchor in Pusan harbour, was the Danish hospital ship *Jutlandia*. Some of the cases of maxillo-facial injuries from Twenty-nine Brigade were treated there.

After the formation of Number One British Commonwealth Division, the medical set-up, instead of having an American MASH support, the division was allocated the Norwegian Hospital, whose establishment was about the same as an American MASH.

X-ray facilities were available at this level. An evacuation system was used where a team of helicopters (attached to either Corps HQ or the MASH) was always available if required, and there was always evacuation to Iwakuni (near Kure, Japan) from the nearest airfield to the front.

Patients were drawn mainly from sick parades, which were fairly large, and these supplied the majority of attendances. Visits were made to units where possible, but operations made these difficult as the units were in the line for the majority of the time.

Medical stores were at Kure and supplies were flown over when required. Early on, certain items were difficult, e.g. methylated spirits; but this was only a temporary shortage. Bottles of local anaesthetic, medicaments, zelex and lysol solutions and phenol were frequently frozen on winter mornings. In general, American space heaters on issue provided adequate comfort, warmth and kept materials in usable form.

AN ADEN EPISODE
[Cpl W. Wilkinson, RADC]

Life under active service conditions in Aden was varied and exhilarating, despite the restrictions imposed by the activities of the dissident terrorists and the summer climate.

From October until April the weather in Aden is one of the most temperate in the world. From April on, however, it becomes unremittingly more oppressive. Late July and August is a period of intense heat (up to 140° F). It is at this time that the usual on-shore breeze ceases. At intervals in its place comes a burning blast from the desert bringing sandstorms which obscure everything to within a few yards in every direction and patients reporting for treatment with sand caked masks to the sweat on their faces.

There was indeed a marked variety in the types of patient who passed through the surgeries. Intelligence agents and undercover men, with .38 revolvers in shoulder holsters, or 7.9 Beretta automatics stuffed in the waistband of trousers under loose-fitting Blue Island shirts. British Service personnel seconded to the Federal Army, Royal Marine Commando, members of the Special Air Service. Once the entire crew of a destroyer which had been forced to decommission because of an intestinal epidemic came; also dissidents from Almansura Prison.

The daily routine was also liable to quick reversals in role. One minute one was assisting in the treatment of a patient, the next riding 'shotgun' in a landrover taking the Senior Dental Officer the twenty-five miles out to Little Aden on an official visit. We would start off through Khormasker, then down the grim 'Murder Mile' of Malla, Sterling at the ready, eyes narrowed against any hostile move or lofted hand grenade.

Frequently spaced along the Malla Mile were troops with rifles at the ready and officers whose hands were never far from their holstered revolvers. When I first arrived in Aden, I walked down to the Crescent shopping area at Steamer Point one Saturday afternoon, and on the opposite side of the road a corporal of the RAF Provost was walking along with his revolver in his hand.

The journey out to Little Aden past Sheikh Othman, the new Federal Capital at Ahalitaid and the massive BP Oil Refinery, takes one through a towering range of eroded mountains uncannily similar in their magnificent desolation to a lunar landscape.

Another role for the RADC NCO was on an armed guard rota which was carried out for six months with the Prince of Wales Own Regiment of Yorkshire, the duties being to protect the Bowling Alley and Open Air Cinema during the evening performance. This guard had been instigated after a grenade had been hurled at the cinema from a nearby Federal Army Compound, a doubtless necessary precaution as on Christmas Eve the evening was rent by the boom of plastic explosives which had been placed under a truck at the other side of the Federal Army Compound.

Access to the Bowling Alley roof was by means of an iron ladder fastened quite closely to the wall. This made the ascent, in heavy combat boots and clutching an SLR up over the top of an overhanging parapet, just a little bit difficult. In point of fact, one NCO fell off the ladder and injured his back and was never thereafter called upon for this duty again.

One of our patients, a Capt. Weldon of the AAC, had attended a certain cocktail party. Both he and his wife were injured and several people killed by an explosive device, planted by a deserting Yemini servant to blow up in their midst. After I had left Aden, tour expired, I learnt with a terrible sense of tragedy and remorse of the death of one of our former patients, the late Lieutenant Watts of the RNF, slain in the infamous Crater Massacre.

The Central Dental Laboratory in Aden was located at the RAF Hospital Steamer Point. In order to prevent delay on the return of repaired dentures we undertook, when necessary, to do this work in our spare time, and sometimes produced temporary spoontype partials until the permanent appliance was available. A Patrol Medic of the Special Air Service Regiment asked the Senior Dental Officer, Major Morrey, for a mouth mirror to assist him in placing temporary dressings in carious teeth when out on patrols. Major Morrey provided a handle for a used mirror-head which was still reasonably operational. It was noted that the SAS Patrol Medic accepted this makeshift instrument with a certain pride in possession.

182

Confrontation in Borneo
Operation 'Hearts and Minds'

Conflict began in late 1962, when a group of local Brunei guerrillas, under the leadership of Azahari and sympathisers to President Sukarno of Indonesia, attempted to capture Andaki Airport (Shell Company) at Seria, north of Brunei Town. They also attempted to blow up some oil installations but this was shortlived as men of the Queen's Own Highlanders and Marine Commandos flew in quickly and shot many of the guerrillas including their leader, Azahari (they were put in gaol in Brunei). At the same time several hundred local inhabitants were rounded up by another group of rebels and two couples from Shell were taken hostage. Operation 'Hearts and Minds', planned to discourage tribal involvement with the insurgents, came into being.

Briefly, during 1963, the SAS operating along the border with Indonesia discovered that there was a need for a dentist among the tribes in the area. It is unlikely that they had ever seen a doctor, never mind a dentist. They put in a request, and as usual in all matters affecting them the Army Medical Services did their best to provide. The AMS was thin on the ground over the whole of Borneo. RADC strength in Brunei was a Captain Gordon on a four month attachment from BMH Singapore. (As far as I know he may have been the whole RADC commitment to Borneo at the time.) The Assistant Director of Medical Services could only offer myself, a Cpl Clerk RAMC, with limited medical knowledge, as his assistant.

Captain Gordon briefed me quickly in matters he wanted me to undertake (sterilisation of instruments, amalgams, bits of kit we would need, a quick run through on an old-fashioned treadle-operated drill, etc.) and we went to Brunei Airstrip where we would emplane.

We flew in a Beaver light aircraft. Aboard were the pilot, Capt. Gordon, two Infantrymen, myself, sacks of mail, stores, and as many loaves of bread (baked on *HMS Eagle* and worth their weight in gold to troops in the jungle) as we were able to squeeze in. Somehow, the Beaver got off the ground, but I noticed that we flew *between* mountains rather than *over* them during the whole seventy mile trip.

We landed at Dario airstrip, which is about two miles inside the imaginary border. Somehow the word had got out, and we were met by scores of Dyak tribespeople, a band, and lots of cheers. Capt. Gordon admitted to being moved, as he was not used to such a welcome – waiting rooms not being noted for good cheer.

As the Dyaks had walked some distance for the event, we had to start treatment there and then, in the Airport Control (a hut). Plans for moving out were put back until the next day. We treated an unknown number of patients and quickly ran out of dental anaesthetic for the cartridge syringe (although we had started with two boxes). Captain Gordon enquired whether the SAS 'medic' had extracted any teeth and was told "scores". He had borrowed a pair of pliers from the crew of a visiting aircraft and used the normal strength local anaesthetic to pull teeth. As Dyaks had just put up with bad teeth before his arrival, the SAS boy was soon established as the dentist. His efforts were appreciated by all but himself. He knew he had no training and wanted to do something better for the tribes. (He inherited all our instruments and some training from Captain Gordon when we left).

We stayed the night at the SAS camp prior to moving off the next day. However, more Dyaks arrived from distant long houses and we had to start late, having stayed to treat them. As we had to arrive by nightfall, our first march was a bit forced. It consisted of a nine-mile yomp along jungle tracks, over a succession of ridges and valleys, rivers, bridges (log and rope), etc. It was very difficult country and the forty pound Bergan we carried caused my shoulders to bleed. Both Captain Gordon and myself were very unfit in those days, definitely not in the same league as the SAS patrol which took us. I suffered cramps, which was relieved by salt tablets.

Immediately on arrival in Pa Mein (I think), we started work again. By this time Captain Gordon had graduated to taking out whole mouthfuls of worn-down stumps. He discovered that the Dyaks had soft jaw bones and was able to extract most teeth by levering them out with an instrument shaped like a mustard spoon (I

184

don't know the correct term for this instrument). All operations took place surrounded by a large audience who were very appreciative and they encouraged the patients noisily by clapping and cheering as we each took a turn. A small boy kept score of teeth pulled by chalking on a wall.

Sterilisation of instruments was a full-time job. The method was boiling in a pot over a wood fire. By this time we were short of any type of anaesthetic as the strong dental local anaesthetic had run out and the normal skin LA was in short supply.

Life became a round of moving from long house to long house, each some miles apart. Patients came from both sides of the border as the tribe did not take notice of this artificial boundary.

The pay-off for our efforts was the long conversations which took place as visiting Dyaks in the long house got into conversation with the SAS who then tapped out messages back to base. The information gleaned was good enough for the Royal Artillery batteries to put down timed interdiction fire on tracks and crossings quite effectively.

We were in the area about two weeks before returning. Several practical lessons had been learned. New ground was broken and the RADC team due to go in (on some occasion in 1964) was better equipped and achieved more.

As far as Capt. Gordon was concerned, it was a rewarding experience as the need was great and the work carried out was intensive. He probably has a total figure he keeps for *The Guinness Book of Records* (teeth pulled). The effect of drugs (aspirin, oral penicillin, etc.) was remarkable on a population totally unused to drugs. The Heath Robinson dental drill was impractical to backpack long distances and was abandoned just prior to take-off.

NB Wartime expedience led to the secondment of the author, WO I. K. Monk LSL RAMC, then as a (Cpl) dental assistant to Captain Gordon, RADC. They were on a short tour from BMH Singapore to Borneo in 1963 during SAS infiltration of the Indonesian Border. They treated Dyaks in Bario and Pa Mein.

Jungle Jim

As Monk states above, a dental team was posted in from Singapore in 1964. Captain James Chalmers-Clark, RADC, a National Service dental officer, spent one year as DO to the British

Commonwealth troops as well as maintaining the 'Hearts and Minds' operation.

Chalmers-Clark describes his practice as covering a vast area including Brunei, Sarawak and Sabah, with a dental unit in each location supported substantially by the local civilian medical services. The team also visited army patrol (company) positions in the jungle with army air support, carrying portable dental material but no drilling equipment.

Some comfort was derived when the REME and RE detachments made good a mobile dental unit recovered from the mud in Kuching.

At every visit to the jungle locations, inquisitive tribesmen – Dyaks and Murats – descended on the dental team. Most of them were treated alongside the troops and scouts back from patrols. Border scouts usually provided an interpreter and sometimes, from the village, an 'untrained' female nurse.

THE FALKLANDS CAMPAIGN

Prologue

For many years Argentina has held claim to the Malvinas which we know better under their rightful name of the Falkland Islands. In 1982 Argentina mounted an invasion to seize and hold the islands. On 2nd April 1982 massive sea and air-borne Argentinian forces overwhelmed the tiny British Garrison, and next day occupied also the associated dependency of South Georgia.

A Task Force was immediately assembled and despatched to the South Atlantic. Over one hundred ships and twenty-eight thousand service personnel were involved. Four RADC dental officers and soldiers were on the strength of either Sixteen Field Ambulance or Two Field Hospital. The Field Ambulance provided second-line medical support to the ground forces while the field hospital gave third-line medical support to the army. The dental officers were employed primarily on resuscitation duties.

After a voyage of eight thousand miles units of the task force first landed on the Falklands during the night of the 20/21 May at San Carlos Bay. A pincer attack was launched against the Argentinian forces in Port Stanley. The northern element of the attack was from Three Commando Brigade, which had to make its way right across the island of East Falkland. Helicopters were invaluable in moving forward artillery and stores, but because of the wet and muddy terrain men had to move on foot. The Royal Marines yomped their way across.

The southern pincer element was made up of units from Five Infantry Brigade. These included One Welsh guards, Two Scots Guards and Sixteen Field Ambulance. They were moved by sea to the south-eastern coast and landed at Bluff Cove. Here, landing craft suffered a devastating aerial bombing attack. Pte K. M. Reeves

RADC survived the attack on Sir Galahad but there were many casualties.

Despite the enormous difficulties they encountered, our forces were able to fight their way to occupy the high ground to the west and south of Port Stanley. By 11th June the Argentinian forces were in an impossible position. They were under constant observation and heavy artillery bombardment. On 14th June 1982 Argentinian resistance collapsed and General Menendez surrendered to the British military commander, Major General (Sir) Jeremy Moore.

A DENTAL OFFICER IN THE FALKLAND ISLANDS
[Lt Col K. A. C. Watt, BDS]

Leaving my normal duties as Dental Officer to the Scottish Infantry Depot (Bridge of Don) on May 12th, 1982, I found myself in the early hours embarking on the *QE2* at Southampton Docks in my operational role of Resuscitation Officer to one of the two Field Surgical Teams (FST), each composed of one surgeon, one anaesthetist, one resuscitation officer, one blood transfusion orderly and four operating theatre technicians, attached to Sixteen Field Ambulance RAMC for operations in the South Atlantic.

The *Queen Elizabeth II*
A familiar role soon presented during the voyage south, as the two other RADC officers and I busied ourselves looking after the dental emergencies among the ship's complement of 4,000 plus. By courtesy of Cunard and *QE2's* hospital staff and I trust, with the subsequent approval of the ship's dental officer, we made full use of the neat dental surgery located within the hospital. Although my records are incomplete, in excess of 124 emergency dental treatments were provided during our seventeen days aboard *QE2*, a high incidence of acute periodontal infections, included pericoronitis, being noted.

Non-dental duties included military and physical training; briefings on intelligence and the Falkland Islands; practice at various stations, such as boat, flying defence and assault and FST training (consisting of lectures and demonstrations to our own and other personnel); plus equipment familiarisation.

Off-duty activities afloat included sleeping, viewing films and videos, reading (especially the *Field Surgery Pocket Book*), socialising, much nervous discussion, a military concert, and enjoying the fine repasts provided in the Queen's Room, occupying seats costing some £100 per day in more normal times. Having called briefly at Freetown on the Sierra Leone Coast on May 18th and crossed the line with much uproarious ceremony, the *QE2* sailed around the waters off Ascension Island for some days to enable transferral of stores and personnel. Amid stringent blackout conditions and with anti-aircraft measures appearing on upper decks, we sailed on southwards amid heavier seas and spectacular icebergs before arriving at South Georgia on May 27th.

Norland

With the *QE2* anchored in Cumberland Bay off Grytviken amid the stark, frozen beauty of South Georgia and in sight of the Argentine submarine and Puma helicopter damaged in the Argentine takeover, our party transferred, via a rusty converted trawler/minesweeper, to the North Sea Ferry MV *Norland* late on May 28th.

San Carlos

First light on June 1st saw us curled up on our bunks in *Norland* wearing full combat kit, tin hat, and life jacket as the ship entered San Carlos water during a red air raid alert. Shortly after a dull dawn we disembarked through a hole in the side of the ship onto a landing craft for the ten-minute trip to our first landfall on the Falkland Islands at Ajax Bay, the site of the Commando Brigade Field Hospital and also a temporary stockade for 400 Argentine POWs.

Having eventually reassembled at the large sheep-shearing sheds in San Carlos Settlement across the bay, another red alert saw some of us diving for cover into prepared trenches. I rapidly sought another hole for myself among the large wool bales when the *Daily Mirror* reporter informed me that my trench had received a direct hit from a bomb two days previously, killing the two Royal Marine occupants.

The deployment of our two FSTs having been arranged in the front garden of the local farm manager's house, our party moved into some spare rooms therein and settled down to await the unloading of our tentage and equipment from two other ferries. Amid continuing red alerts and a stand-to to face a possible Argentine parachute drop,

190

we proceeded to dig our own trenches in increasingly cold and wet conditions. We got to know our hosts, the Short family, who proved very enthusiastic, kind and hospitable, despite the problems we caused to their critical water supplies.

Our equipment having been landed, the FSTs were ordered on June 7th to embark on the RFA *Sir Galahad* for an overnight move to Fitzroy, some fourteen miles from Stanley, to set up a Forward Surgical Centre.

Sir Galahad

We sailed in the early hours of June 8th, much later than scheduled. After a pleasant dinner and evening rounded off with the unaccustomed luxury shower and a bunk, the *Sir Galahad* arrived off Fitzroy as a beautiful red dawn broke. Only one pontoon assembly (Mexiflote) and one landing craft were available for disembarking the large number of troops aboard, and both of these were already part loaded with stores. In the event, after lunch, the first and only party to disembark was the command party element of Sixteen Field Ambulance plus my own FST. Some minutes after landing and 'tabbing' to our new position, the Argentine air attack on the *Sir Galahad* and *Sir Tristram* occurred, and within a further twenty minutes the first casualties started arriving at our position ashore in Fitzroy settlement. One hundred and thirty-five casualties, mostly burns, were treated with dressings, morphia and IV fluids in our hurriedly-improvised facility, prior to being evacuated to the hospital ship SS *Uganda*.

Two further air attacks were made on our area that afternoon, the latter one inspiring a spectacular deterrent show of defensive fireworks, but fortunately no further casualties occurred.

Three members of Sixteen Field Ambulance were killed on the *Sir Galahad* but fortunately no members of our FSTs or the RADC had been injured, although all survivors were severely shaken. As the majority of our personal equipment and all FST equipment had, however, been destroyed, the FSTs were evacuated to Ajax Bay the next day via a fast low-flying Sea King helicopter, after a bitterly cold and exposed night at Fitzroy.

British Assault on Stanley

Amid recurring red alerts and two exploded bombs at Ajax Bay the personnel of our two FSTs were reformed, and Royal Navy surgical equipment cannibalised, to enable my FST to move forward again to Fitzroy on June 11th, in readiness for the imminent final British assault towards Stanley. The attacks started that night and were continued on the night of June 13th. From the time of the arrival of the first Casevac helicopters before first light on June 12th, the Forward Surgical Centre at Fitzroy was kept busy with battle casualties, both British and Argentine, until late on June 15th. During this period I attempted to make myself useful in a Resuscitation Department of six stretcher bays where I worked with a very able and experienced team from 1 Parachute FST processing casualties, after resuscitation, out to two operating tables or for further evacuation.

My impressions of that traumatic period are largely the extremely impressive demeanour, bearing courage and dignity of the sometimes horribly wounded soldiers.

Following the Argentine surrender, we were afforded some time in Fitzroy to reflect on our experiences and to take regular walks along cliffs past the hulks of *Sir Tristram* and the still burning *Sir Galahad*.

Stanley

Moving by Chinook helicopter to Stanley on June 22nd, we rejoined our companion FST which was already in residence providing surgical cover at Stanley Hospital. Finding ourselves therefore redundant, we proceeded for R&R first to the BR Ferry MV *St Edmund* and then to MV *Fort Toronto*, a superb and hospitable Canadian Pacific water tanker whose cargo was guaranteed to have been passed by everybody on board.

Homecoming

Leaving one FST and two dental officers (one RADC, one RAF) in Stanley Hospital, I commenced the long journey back to the UK in considerably less style than I had left, via some hair-raising exploits on small boats in rough seas, up and down long rope ladders slung over cavernous ships' sides, to be followed by crushingly uncomfortable long hours in an RAF Hercules aircraft.

A FIELD AMBULANCE IN THE FALKLANDS WAR
[Major G. K. Long]

By the time Sixteen Field Ambulance embarked on the liner *QE2* on May 12th I had been with the unit as dental officer for over eighteen months and had travelled extensively with them on many exercises. These brief notes were extracted from my 'war diary' kept daily from May 19th until I embarked on the *SS Uganda* for the return home on August 13th.

After landing at the San Carlos bridgehead on the 1st June and settling in, a few days were spent while the brigade was reorganised and readied for its move east towards Port Stanley and its eventual recapture. I was included in the Advance Dressing Station (ADS) and there was much talk about us making an early move from San Carlos. On 5th June the ADS, about thirty strong, were warned for a move to Fitzroy Cove. However, after we had all waited for most of the day in the rain and mud around San Carlos jetty, the plan was changed and we all returned to our digs.

The following day saw us waiting on a helipad again, in continuous rain and high winds but not so much mud. This time we had divided our kit and men into three sticks, each of which would be carried by a Sea King helicopter. Well, after two hours one Sea King arrived and lifted off twelve men but no kit, so the rest of us waited patiently. By this time all of us were drenched despite wearing a complete set of water proofs. Finally after nearly a four hour wait, flying was shut down due to worsening conditions.

Plans were quickly changed to allow us to move to Fitzroy by sea and as darkness fell we set to, moving all the ADS kit the half mile back to San Carlos jetty before cross loading it over one landing craft to another. Finally we set off to sail out to the RFA *Sir Tristram* moored in Falkland Sound. Once there, we onloaded all the kit into the hold of the ship before we could attempt to dry the kit out and find a bed for the night.

Next morning, just as the dawn broke, *Sir Tristram* moored in Fitzroy Cove. At the stern of the ship, kit and vehicles were being unloaded onto landing craft through the large near door, and I went along to see how the unloading of the ADS kit was progressing. I was somewhat shocked to find us moored in a small inlet surrounded by completely flat land, while clearly visible about six miles away were the range of mountains around Port Stanley, Mounts Kent and Challenger, and the Twin Sisters. It was general knowledge that the Argentinian observation posts were situated there. The weather that day was unforgettable; a clear blue sky with no clouds and bright sunshine with perfect visibility, a complete contrast to everything that had gone before.

Ashore, I was relieved to find that our twelve colleagues had arrived safely the previous evening and were sharing the settlement with Two Para. A small queue had already formed outside the village shop which was doing a roaring trade. The couple who ran the shop later left the Falklands at the earliest opportunity and returned to Belfast, which they felt was much safer. Several hours work saw our tentage up and all the kit installed and we were ready for business. We sat back to await the arrival of the field ambulance main body expected the following day.

As has been well documented, next day, the 8th June, the RFA *Sir Galahad* sailed into Fitzroy Sound on another beautifully clear sunny day and, following several delays in unloading, eventually formed a perfect target for the Argentinian jet planes which bombed both it and the *Sir Tristram*. Ashore this was watched with a mixture of surprise and horror which lasted about fifteen minutes, before the first casualties were brought the half mile from the beach to our treatment area. What followed was two hours of frenzied activity in which 135 casualties, including seventy stretcher cases, were treated and evacuated by a very small body of men, helped towards the end by an increasing number of field ambulance medics who had got off the ship unhurt. Tragically our second-in-command and two of our soldiers were killed in the attack.

There was little time to recover from this disaster because by now the familiar cry of 'Air Raid Red' rang out. Having been instructed not to dig in until told, we had no trenches to go to, so I retired to the safety of a thick hedge about a quarter of a mile away from the settlement. Before long, six Argentinian jet planes were seen circling the area. Every so often a ground-to-air missile would be fired at them, most of these tracing loops in air without finding a target. Later we heard that most of these jets had been shot down while attacking the Scots Guards at Bluff Cove further down the coast. However, one got through to Fitzroy and flew very low over our Dressing Station, possibly no more than fifty feet above the ground. As it came within range the small arms fire from the whole of Two Para and all the other troops was unleashed on the Skyhawk. There followed a most awesome display of firepower with the whole sky was lit up by red tracer bullets. The jet banked and weaved its way through all this, thankfully without dropping any of its bombs. It was later shot down by a Rapier battery as it returned home. After that brief moment of excitement we were brought back to earth with a bump. All our kit on the ships had been lost, all people on the ship had lost all their personal possessions apart from what they stood up in. The Advanced ADS was virtually stripped bare after the treatment provided earlier. For the first time I thought that perhaps I would not get back to the UK alive.

The next two days were a period of rapid reorganisation, resupply and reinforcements, which rendered us operational again. Survivors from the ship returned after rest and recuperation (R&R) and rekitting. Trenches were dug, the pessimists among us digging some marvellously deep and complicated earth works. I even managed to find a square of carpet to line the seat of my trench. Shift systems were set up, eight hours on, eight off, as we had practised many times on exercise. We carried on seeing a trickle of casualties and the daily medical and dental sick.

The start of the final battle to retake Port Stanley officially began at 2359 hours on 11th June. The distant thumps and flashes of artillery shells could be seen and heard in the early hours of the following morning. The first battle casualties began arriving at about 0730, slow at first but increasing towards midday, as the daylight increased. The next few days seemed to blur together, working eight hours on, eight hours off, eating three meals during the nine daylight hours and treating streams of casualties, both British and Argentinian following the separate battles during those days and nights.

Another memorable moment came early in the afternoon of the 15th June with the radio message that our troops had reached Stanley and that a ceasefire had been announced. I had been suturing the lips and chin of a Scots guardsman at the time. There was a great shout of delight in our treatment tent and the patients cheered up enormously. The following weeks were best forgotten in my view. A rapidly decreasing work load and with the increasing boredom, frustration and disillusionment set in. Return to the UK seemed unlikely for the foreseeable future and it looked as though our stay might be for a further six months. The weather rapidly deteriorated as the winter set in with snow, freezing cold, and high winds making life very uncomfortable at times. The gloom was lifted eventually when it was arranged for us to return home on the hospital ship *SS Uganda*. The remaining members of the unit boarded the one Chinook helicopter at Fitzroy and flew to Port Stanley, a very exciting journey seemingly about ten feet off the ground while the pilot ate his sandwiches in one hand and steered with the other.

SOME REFLECTIONS ON OPERATION CORPORATE

[Major J. F. Aitken]

In March 1982 when I attended Exercise 'Top Cat', prior to starting my year's attachment to Two Field Hospital, the Commanding Officer, in his opening address, lamented the fact that the unit had not been called into action for many years. Little did he know what the future had in store or the elements of his command. I thought it a possibility that I might find myself in such a situation, nevertheless I was still surprised to find myself on board the *QE2* about to set sail for some pink dot on the atlas. After all, unlike those members of the 'teeth arms' who spend considerable time training for war, ours is a peacetime occupation and to suddenly find oneself being issued with a pistol and live ammunition does tend to come as a bit of a shock.

At least a year later what does one remember? For those lucky enough to remain unscathed, memories fade quickly, stories improve for the telling and become more embellished as time goes by. Some memories stick – the overwhelming send-off from Southampton, the first view of the Falklands as we disembarked from the *Norland*, my first encounter with a casualty, or those 'magic' bread buns made by one of the two field cooks in Stanley Hospital.

How extraordinary to be going off to war on one of the world's most luxurious cruise liners. True, nearly all the trimmings had been removed, but basically she was still the same ship that people had paid thousands of pounds on which to cruise. The whole voyage down to South Georgia had an unreal feel about it. To sit in the Queen's Grill and watch soldiers pounding round the decks, or the

Gurkhas, blindfolded and in full foul weather gear, make way round the ship – how difficult it was to relate it all to that mythical island so far away.

Frustration increased, tempers became short and frayed. What were we going to do? Were we going to get there on time? Was anybody *actually* interested in the medical teams? We began to wonder. Then there were all those wonderful stories about us being 'discovered' by a Russian trawler in Freetown and of *Canberra* armed with Exocet looking for us. One day we were sunk, or as one of our anaesthetists put it, "It's not true that the *QE2* has been sunk, isn't it?" We wondered what was happening to our families at home. All the thoughts that must have passed through the minds of thousands in similar situations before us passed through ours.

Reality began to creep in as we sailed further south. It became colder. General purpose machine guns and blow pipes appeared on the upper decks. Assault stations started. Even that didn't go well for us – we actually made it into a helicopter on our third attempt. Can't say the idea of being transhipped by helicopter did anything for our morale. Particularly as by then we had heard the news of the SAS helicopter loss.

Finally we arrived at night in the bay off Grytvinken to see in the gloom the lights of *Canberra* and *Norland* and discover some North Sea trawlers. The following day the sun rose and the mist cleared to reveal a tremendous panorama. That day was to be a formidable example of the 'hurry up and wait' syndrome but eventually we made it on to the *Norland*. During the day survivors from the bombed *Ardent* and *Antelope* had embarked on the *QE2*. How odd it was to realise that they were on the way home, that their war was over. *They* had survived. Would *we*?

On the *Norland* things began to change. The news of Goose Green came through. Pete Coombes (I'll tell you when it hurts, lads) was no longer able to have us jumping up and down on the decks. The ship seemed to be littered with green-looking Gurkhas clutching paper bags. The mornings started with music blaring over the tannoy. "Here comes the sun" and "Ra, Ra, hello, happy Gurkhas" – quite horrendous. Of course, the *Norland* had been in and out before and the crew were credited with bringing down a plane. So it was nothing new to them. The RN 2IC in fact gave running commentaries during air raids.

So we arrived in 'bomb alley' and disembarked. Beautiful day – thought we were supposed to be landing during the dark! Sure it's not Scotland? Wrong beach of course, we were supposed to be over the other side of the bay.

San Carlos settlement found some of use accommodated in the home of a farm manager, others in the village hall. Not long after our arrival we had experienced our first 'Air Raid Red', so our first priority was to dig a trench. Good grief, what hard work, and what a superb residence we had by the time we had finished. A few days later we were warned that the Argentinians were going to counter-attack the following day. At dawn the next morning we were to be found crouching in our trenches, pistols at the ready, waiting for the expected airborne invasion. We were finally driven out by the noise of the marines quite unconcernedly going off to breakfast. The air was thick with rumours and stories. Never mind, we were dry and reasonably comfortable, unlike the majority out on the hills.

The *Sir Galahad* incident left us slightly bemused, short of kit and saddened at the terrible loss of life and injuries. Feelings ran high. For the first time as a unit we were split up – some of us going to Ajax Bay, others to Fitzroy. More equipment was gathered up and we were back in business just a few hours before the deadline. Fear of the unknown is usually far worse than the real thing, and it was with considerable apprehension that I, a complete novice, stood around in the resuscitation area, hopefully with an air of confidence, waiting for the first casualties. We were among the experts who had been there from the start and were under their watchful and initially resentful eyes. One of their teams had already been away for eight months, having been diverted on their way back from the Gulf. Once the first batch of casualties had arrived all other thoughts were forgotten. I was amazed by their condition and cheerfulness. The next few days passed by quickly and suddenly it was all over – Stanley had been retaken. After that, it was just a matter of tidying up and waiting for the order to move. A few more casualties still trickled in. It is hard to forget the rather pathetic sight of the young Argentinian conscripts with self-inflicted injuries who were brought in from West Falklands. Apparently they had hoped to be taken into hospital where there was more food.

The other half of the building started to fill up with Argentinian prisoners. It seemed rather poetic justice that they should share a room with one of their own unexploded bombs. It was quite amusing to see them shepherded around wearing Canberra luggage labels waiting to be shipped off. The contrast between their officers and other ranks was quite surprising. The officers still had their creature comforts – radios, cameras, typewriters, etc. – and were clean and tidy.

It was decided that we would move round to Stanley. The following evening we embarked on the *Elk* for the trip. The next morning we disembarked and made our way to the hospital to discover that Two Field Hospital had arrived the same day. It was good to be able to pay a visit to *SS Uganda*, the hospital ship. We were most impressed by the set-up and the tremendous work they had done. We were overwhelmed by their hospitality, and the return flight remains somewhat hazy. Much to our embarrassment we found ourselves in charge of a prisoner – an Argentinian dental officer – whom we were to deliver to the hospital. Fortunately he did not run off and we arrived back safely with a certain amount of a well-known tincture. I had also managed to come away clutching a bag of tinned haggis and a side of smoked salmon – *Uganda* had been celebrating a halfway to Burns Night supper. They were superb.

Stanley was still littered with piles of ammunition, equipment and abandoned vehicles. Souvenir hunting was a major pastime. It was said that a certain guards officer tried to ship out a vehicle for use on his farm back home.

Peacetime soldiering returned and it started to snow in Stanley. It was time to go home. On 4th July just as the light was fading a lucky few of us left Stanley on the first stage of the homeward journey. In the early hours of the 6th July we slid quietly into RAF Lyneham and from there on to Aldershot, where I discovered that my wife had been misdirected and was waiting for me at Brize Norton.

I had only been away for eight weeks but it seemed like half a lifetime. To think what it must have been like during the last world war for those who were away for years and for the people they left at home.

IN THE FALKLANDS WITH A FIELD HOSPITAL RAMC

[Lt Col C. H. Lee]

I went to the South Atlantic in 1982 as a member of the advance party of Two Field Hospital RAMC, which was part of a large mixed unit that was to deal with the organisation of prisoners.

The unexpected experience started for me when I was telephoned one afternoon in May. A trip to Aldershot for a briefing and to collect field kit followed and then I was on seventy-two hour standby. It therefore came as a surprise to be telephoned at 2300 hours on 2nd June and told to be in Aldershot at 1200 hours the next day.

I met Cpl Joe Green and Cpl Mark Adams, the other Dental Corps members of the unit for the first time. On the 6th June we paraded at Two Field Hospital, went to Brize Norton by bus, and were then issued with our weapons. There we met up with other elements of our unit – Royal Corps of Transport, Intelligence Corps, Catering Corps, there being one hundred and ten personnel in all.

The flight to Ascension Island in a VC10 was pleasant and took eleven and a half hours, including a one hour fuel stop in Dakar in Senegal where we were not allowed off the aircraft. We wondered what to expect in Ascension. Our experience there made us feel that it must be one of the worst places in the world. Arriving at 2300 hours the weather was humid with a steady drizzle and we were loaded into trucks for a four mile trip to English Bay. This turned out to be a tented camp where everything was covered with thick Ascension dust. To make matters worse, all our identical kit was tipped out of the truck onto the wet earth and had to be sorted out in the dark.

We were glad to leave the next morning, and although it was known that we were going south by ship there was speculation as to which one. When we heard the name *Dumbarton Castle*, it conjured up visions of a cruise liner, but our hopes were dashed when we heard that *HMS Dumbarton Castle* was a 1,500 ton North Sea protection vessel. As we prepared for our helicopter trip to the ship we were not aware of another experience to come when we were lowered by rope to the small helicopter deck of the ship. Baggage had to be sorted out again from a large pile on the deck.

Conditions on board were cramped, as the ship's company were forty and we were 110 extra. The twelve day trip was no holiday cruise and the rough seas affected the small ship badly. People had trouble staying in their seats or camp beds and the amount of china broken was enormous. Shaving day after day while hanging on to a water pipe and wedging one's feet was also entertaining. We passed the time with endless videos, a practice shoot over the stern, and when the weather was too bad for deck use we practised 'action stations' in our anti-flash gear. When we were in the Falklands exclusion zone there were one or two real 'action stations' but as the lower part of the ship was full of ammunition and the helicopter deck was stacked with missiles and aviation fuel, one wondered what would happen to a ship this size if it were hit!

We were able to get very little information on what was happening in the Falklands. After we heard of the ceasefire we were told that we would go into Port Stanley and come alongside the British Rail ferry *MV St Edmund*, which towered above us. They lowered a lifeboat to our level and all our kit was spilled into it, again to be deposited in a heap. We stayed aboard the *St Edmund* for a few days, commuting ashore to the hospital. The Scots Guards were on board recovering from their experience.

It became apparent that the prisoner situation was rapidly being resolved and that they were being repatriated as soon as possible. Only the officers and professional engineers were retained. Our unit therefore was split up and the Two Field Hospital element took over part of the small civilian hospital for a military wing. Stanley was in a considerable mess when we went ashore, with live ammunition, abandoned kit, food and filth everywhere. The change that had been brought about when we left three months later was enormous. In the early days, when everyone turned their hand to anything that needed doing, Cpl Green helped in the wards and Cpl Adams assisted sorting out the large quantity of Argentinian medical stores.

During July the civilian dentist went back to the UK on leave and we were kept busy throughout, with army, RAF, and civilian patients ashore and Naval and Merchant Navy patients coming off the many ships that were calling in Port Stanley. There was quite a lot of denture work to do and Cpl Green was kept busy, also becoming a specialist in repairing spectacles. We were kept more fully occupied than most, so there was little time for joy riding. Visits to Naval ships in port and the Hospital Ship *SS Uganda* made a pleasant change. Arriving on board *SS Uganda* in combat kit, one felt rather out of place when being entertained in the ornate dining-room with printed menus and uniformed waiters, but we were grateful to obtain a supply of tobacco and spirits.

The return journey was by Hercules to Ascension Island, which took twelve hours. Not as bad as my successor, who had to make three trips because of bad weather, but long enough to prevent one being concerned about a long aeroplane journey in future. We flew back to the UK in a VC10, but just as we thought we were home we flew to Germany and spent a night fogbound there – which at least did enable us to buy some wine.

THE GULF WAR

Prologue

At 0200 hours on 2nd August 1990 Iraqi forces attacked Kuwait, and within twenty-four hours had occupied most of the country. Lieutenant-Colonel J. Q. Anderson, RADC, was attached to Operation Granby, a British operational contingent within the UN forces. He describes the Defence Dental Service deployment in the Gulf as follows.

...On 9th August RAF aircraft were to be deployed in support of Desert Shield, arriving in Dharan from Cyprus two days later. Hectic activities to make air crew and supporting ground staff dentally fit was seen in RAF dental centres across Cyprus, UK and RAF (G). Medical support for this was to be provided by a hundred bed response from Twenty-Two Field Hospital and the two 'purpose built' Medical Support Troops (MST) Alpha and Bravo. The MSTs were effectively self contained in surgical teams complete with their own transport, equipment, and nursing and clerical staff.

A dental officer was deployed with each MST, dual-roled as CASO and GDDO. Additionally MST Bravo had a DCA employed as a BTA. The Twenty-Two Field Hospital deployed its dental department with GDDO, SPDO DTech, and DCA. The hospital deployed to Bahrain in immediate support of the RAF squadron at Muharraq and as third-line facility for the squadrons at Dhahran and Tobuk where MSTs Alpha and Bravo deployed, respectively.

The Royal Naval Armilla Patrol, already on station in the Gulf area, had its Squadron Dental Officer embarked as a matter of routine. Maritime medical support to the reinforced Armilla Patrol was enhanced by the conversion of the aviation training ship RFA *Argus* to a hundred bed primary casualty receiving ship (PCRS) which included a GDDO, SPDO and two DSAs amongst its compliment.

On Friday 14th September it was announced that Britain would commit ground forces to the Middle East in the form of the Seven Armd Bde Group. Medical Support was provided by One Armd Fd Amb. (reinforced by Four Armd Fd Amb.) deployed as two medical squadrons and Twenty-Four (Sirmob) Fd Amb. Third-line hospital support was provided by the four hundred bed Thirty-Three Field Hospital (CMH). All three units were reinforced by extra RADC personnel in both dental and ancillary war roles. While units were preparing to leave BAOR and UK, Army Dental Centres repeated the RAF experience of a month earlier with the extra complication of wholesale redeployment of dental teams to fill shortfalls and reinforce garrisons with troops earmarked for the Gulf.

On 22nd November the two hundred bed Thirty-Two Field Hospital (BMH *Hanover*) deployed into the Forward Force Maintenance Area (FFMA) in support of the division and reinforcements to Twenty-Two Fd Hosp brought it also up to two hundred beds as it moved forward to Bahrain into the FFMA alongside Thirty-Two Field Hospital. Thirty-Three Field Hospital was reinforced and expanded to six hundred beds to be retitled Thirty-Three General (Surg.) Hospital and remained at Al Jubail in the Force Maintenance Area (FMA). Two hundred and five (Scottish) General Hospital deployed to Riyadh as a six hundred bed facility and Number Four RAF War Hospital (Ely) replaced Twenty-Two Field Hospital in Bahrain as a hundred bed unit.

Further hospital support was provided by a two hundred bed Norwegian Field Hospital – *Normedcoy* – deployed in the FMA in support of Thirty-Three General Hospital, and the hundred bed One (CDN) Field Hospital colocated with Thirty-Two Field Hospital in the FFMA. A Rumanian Field Hospital also arrived in theatre but was held in reserve. All the above units deployed with dental staff in both dental and ancillary roles. Medical resupply was provided through Eighty-Four FMED which deployed with ten D Hyg and nine DCAs in BTA/med storemen roles. Mention should also be made of the Swedish hospital deployed in support of the Allies and of the medical personnel provided by the New Zealand Army.

Other personnel in the KTO were one Dental Support Officer as watch-keeper with Med Branch HQ (UK) Div and two RAF GDDOs as Flt Comds with Number One Aeromedical Evacuation Squadron. Allocation of Dental Service personnel to units and the overall numbers deployed in each primary role, with a glossary, is shown at the end of this narrative.

In addition to their primary roles many staff undertook secondary tasks such as NCB decontamination teams, helicopter handler, med. storeman, assistant medical officer, mortuary assistant, intelligence officer, R & R officer, and many others.

In-theatre dental cover was provided to land and air forces continuously from 20th August 1990 to 11th July 1991: a total of 326 days. At sea dental cover was provided by the GDDO of the Armilla Patrol and the SPDO and GDDO on RFA *Argus*.

Dental casualties (on land) averaged 0.17 per 100 men per day, however amongst TA and reservists this figure was almost quadrupled.

In total approximately 6,000 British Servicemen in KTO became dental casualties during this period by the dental centre set up in Al Jubail to support the Logistic Support Group (LSG) during the recovery phase. Although most units managed to submit accurate treatment returns, an attempt to collate morbidity figures was less successful with only seventy to eighty percent of returns fully complete. Nevertheless some significant trends are revealed.

- Over 40% of dental casualties during deployment and hostilities were presented complaining of pain, compared to only 12% during the recovery phase.
- Of 1,782 reported cases complaining of pain during deployment and hostilities, 340 (19.1%) were due to pericoronitis. Of the 76 cases seen during the recovery phase, 15 (19.7%) were due to pericoronitis.
- 56% of the cases of pericoronitis prior to the ceasefire gave histories of the previous problems, compared to only 27% during the recovery period.
- 1,229 cases of failed/broken/lost restorations were reported.
- 216 failed crowns and bridges were reported.
- Over 650 teeth were extracted and 2,334 restorations placed.

Equipment to deal with the problems described was the subject of much discussion. The 1987 pattern dental equipment set was deployed universally as part of medical unit PUEs. Designed to provide emergency treatment during a short but very intense conflict in NW Europe, this equipment was soon found to be wanting.

Indeed, these limitations in the field equipment had been identified some time before the Gulf crisis, and a few new units had been on trial. Parts of four of these found their way into the KTO to provide enhanced facilities in a few locations. More units were ordered, however only a few ancillary pieces arrived in theatre before the cessation of hostilities, due to the time taken for manufacturers to produce the equipment and the transit time from the UK.

A tri-service committee is considering field equipment at the moment so that any future deployment may be better equipped from the start.

In conclusion, despite weakness in some areas, Operation Granby demonstrated the dental service's ability to respond to the challenge of its dental and ancillary war roles, both those anticipated and a few which were not!

Despite the high levels of dental fitness achieved prior to deployment, nearly fifteen percent of the force was presented with a dental problem, more than justifying the need for a field dental service. The Gulf showed the following quote from the British Dental Association to be as true now as when it was written seventy-three years ago:

> Events have shown beyond all doubt that a modern army cannot operate effectively without an appropriate dental establishment organised and equipped for its special needs.

Fig 1 Operation Granby – Primary Roles of Defence Dental
Personnel in the Kuwait Theatre of Operations (KTO)

Officers		*Soldiers*	
CASO	27	BTA	27
GDDO	24 (i)	DCA	24 (i)
SPDO	9	CDC	9
Treatments	4	Clk	4
Sqn OC	3	DHyg	3
Resuscitation	2	DTech	2
Flt Comd	2	CMT	2
Hosp 21C	1	Liaison	1
Triage	1		1
NBC Officer	1		1
Watchkeeper	1		1
TOTALS	75		75

Notes: (i)   1 Canadian, 1 New Zealand and 1 Norwegian GDDO
        (ii) 1 Canadian and 1 Norwegian DCA
        (iii) 1 New Zealand Dhyg.

Glossary

CASO = Combat Anaesthesia Support Officer
GDDO = General Duty Dental Officer
SPDO = Specialist Dental Officer
BTA   = Blood Transfusion Assistant
CDC   = Chemical Decontamination Centre
CMT   = Combat Medical Technician
FMA   = Force Maintenance Area
PUES = Prestocked Unit Equipments

AN ARMY DENTIST AT WAR IN THE GULF

[Major E. B. Carmichael, MBE, RADC]

Major Ewan Carmichael, RADC, a dental surgeon, commanded B Squadron of One Armoured Field Ambulance RAMC during the Gulf War in 1991. His squadron supported the British Artillery Group during the ground war and saw service in Saudi Arabia, Iraq, and Kuwait.

...When Kuwait was invaded by Iraq forces on 2nd August 1990, I knew instinctively that I would become involved in some way and it came as no surprise when the call to arms was received. I had already been commanding a squadron of Four Armoured Field Ambulance for two years and I felt confident that I understood my role and knew my men. Now we were to reinforce One Armoured Field Ambulance and put our training to the test as Eight Squadron of that unit.

My task was to ensure that the squadron was at the peak of readiness in time for the start of hostilities, and my major concern was how to keep so many adult men occupied and cheerful in the potentially hostile and featureless environment of the desert.

The first aim was achieved by training hard by day and night, the second by paying constant attention to the men's welfare and for the provision of imaginative (hopefully) leisure and sporting pursuits. It would have been too easy to work remorselessly and become stale before the kick-off. It was vital to maintain a high level of discipline and this was enforced intelligently by all ranks from the very beginning. By the start of the war the training, attention to detail, and the discipline had all contributed to a remarkable sense of morale within the squadron.

Our role was in support of the Artillery Group. One of my tasks was to plan and develop procedures for the evacuation and care of wounded during the artillery raids. These raids were to be part of the 'softening up' process prior to breaching the main Iraqi defences. We deployed into the Saudi-Iraqi border area on the night of 14/15th February 1991. The first raid took place a few days later, and one was acutely aware of an almost overwhelming sense of anticipation. Would we be up to the job? Were my plans sound? At the same time, however, I was conscious of, and strengthened by, the rich heritage of courage in the face of adversity within the Army Medical Services.

The squadron crossed the border into Iraq on 24th February 1991 in order to support the breaching operation. This was achieved ahead of schedule, allowing us to transit the breach and follow a series of assaults on enemy positions within Iraq.

On one occasion, in the dark, one of my sections recovered casualties from an area strewn with unexploded munitions. The Section Medical officer earned herself a Mention in Despatches that night.

At times the weather, with its thunder and leaden skies, would have made a most impressive backdrop for a production of *Macbeth*. That and the constant harassment provided by the bombs, shells and rockets of the allied forces, contributed to the enemy's poor morale. Whether injured or not, they were all in such a pitiful condition that even the hardest British hearts were soon softened.

Our entry into Kuwait took place after a long drive through thousands of what can only be described as military refugees who were begging for food and water. It was uplifting to see our soldiers pause briefly to share out their own precious rations before rushing to catch up.

Further advances were only halted on the announcement of a ceasefire. Our war was over and we had suffered no losses. The squadron was ordered to a new position near the Kuwait–Basra highway from where several teams were despatched to Kuwait City to support the potentially hazardous business of bomb disposal there.

The withdrawal phase was perhaps the most frustrating as every man eagerly awaited his return home. In reality, the wait was not too protracted as we were kept busy with essential post-operational administration; discipline and morale within the squadron remained exemplary to the very end.

It was a great privilege to work with such a professional team. Indeed, teamwork was the key to the success of the whole operation.

Operation Granby: the Interesting Bits

Crunch, crunch, chomp, bang, thud. Mantis swallowed the paté and smiled apprehensively. "It don't quite taste the same with compo biscuits, sir."

"Ten minutes to go. I suppose I'd better look lively. Warn the boys!"

I walked across to the Spartan where Commander Artillery had his tactical headquarters. The walk was careful and deliberate, planned to conceal my mounting excitement. In about ten minutes all hell would break loose in the first British artillery raid.

We had come a long way since our first pioneering steps into the desert. Dressing Station One Bravo had been evolved and grown since October 1990. We now numbered 290 all ranks (of nineteen cap badges). We had kept ourselves fit and disease-free through the mind-numbing months of preparation. We became skilled in desert navigation, and if any of our sixty-six vehicles became bogged-in (à la *Ice Cold in Alex*), we now knew all the tricks of the trade needed to extract them.

Christmas had come and had been duly celebrated, leaving only a grim determination to get out and 'finish the job'. In common with our brethren in the hospitals, we had sweated anxious hours away in the knowledge that Scud missiles were airborne. Indeed, we had seen them destroyed.

10 Minutes	…and counting… the disputed zone between Iraq and Saudi Arabia. Spread around are the guns and rocket launchers of two heavy artillery regiments.
9 Minutes	The gunners' mission is to fire into the enemy's depth to disrupt his communications and reinforcement potential.
8 Minutes	On completion of the fire mission, the regiments will hurtle through this rendezvous.
7 Minutes	Our job: to scrape casualties off the passing armour and then 'bug out' ourselves.
6 Minutes	A few kilometres behind me, a 'light dressing station' poised to provide a full range of resuscitative measures.

5 Minutes	10 kilometres further back, the rest of our squadron is providing a reserve in case any of us are killed.
4 Minutes	The threat of counter battery fire is very real – tighten chin strap on helmet.
3 Minutes	Offer up a quick prayer (most sincere).
2 Minutes	Remember to look cheerful.
1 Minute	Silence... and then, of all things, a lark rising.
R Hour	All hell *did* indeed break loose as several MLRS batteries were released at once. It was a truly awe-inspiring sight.

After a few minutes, several grey-orange blossoms flowered to our north. I turned to the Squadron Leader of the Queen's Dragoon Guards Recce Squadron beside me and, summing up as much sang-froid as possible, drawled, "By God, sir, that's incoming fire."

He was well-versed in the story of the Battle of Waterloo, especially the part where the Duke of Uxbridge loses his leg and was able to reply in Wellington terms, "By God, sir, so it is!"

Thankfully, the rogue Iraqi battery was silenced almost as soon as it had unmasked.

The return of our own batteries through the RV was rapid but controlled. Although the order had been issued that there was to be a minimum number of men on all gun positions, it had been disregarded. The guns thundered past with what appeared to be 110% manning. No one wanted to be left behind.

On eliciting that there had been no casualties, we were ourselves then able to make good our own escape. We later learned that at least one enemy position had been destroyed, possibly with up to 300 casualties. It was a sobering and somewhat saddening time.

The raids carried on for the next few days. Sometimes it was the turn of my Squadron 2ic and Liaison officer to win their spurs at the RV. Apart from broadening their experience so that, if needs must, they could step into my shoes, it also allowed me to concentrate on the plans for the next major task – the medical support to the Breach Fire Plan.

At this time, the nights were punctuated with various alarms; the high explosions caused by Fuel Air Explosive, a most exciting alarm mission just to our north and long bursts of heavy calibre machine gunfire which caused us to stand-to for a considerable period one

212

night. At his time the Americans near us had lost several APCs, at night, in minor excursions by Iraqis in company strength.

G-Day, the day of the start of the invasion proper, was meant to see a series of divisionary attacks with the Allies' main assault commencing on G+1. Astonishingly, American progress caused all the plans to be brought forward. Hastily, Order Groups were convened. I barely had time to assemble the whole squadron and finally unveil the plans which had so far only been revealed in outline. The orders were illustrated with a huge burning sand model which hopefully fixed the battle dispositions in everyone's mind.

At 1130 hours on G-Day we drove north a few kilometres and became the first British medical installation to enter Iraq.

The Dressing Station was soon ensconced between the approach lanes to the proposed site of the breach (the main enemy defences being set back from the *de facto* border). Our entrenchments were, at this stage, occupying more and more of our attention. The sobering news that a minor enemy minefield lay only 200m to our north discouraged evening strolls.

The breaching operation was completed with such rapidity that we were able to transit the breach early. The Dressing Station was opened on the far side just in time to support Seven Armoured Brigade's breakout. We witnessed some desultory incoming shell fire to our north.

The night of G+1 saw Captain Mike England RAMC win a well-earned mention in Despatches as he led his section through a field of unexploded bomblets in the dark to rescue several allied casualties. At this time our sister squadron had its only fatality due to the same devices. My CO called me on the secure radio to warn me that he had blown the front wheels of his landrover on the said bomblets. A further advance in the dark was rather like Russian roulette with the squadron deployed in line astern, every driver peering through the gloom praying that he was exactly in the tracks of the vehicle in front.

A subsequent move brought us into the embarrassing position of taking prisoners ourselves. Although medical units are not meant to indulge in such actions, there really was no option but to disarm a few enemy who appeared as we occupied our new position. They were treated firmly but also with kindness. My emotions were, in turn, excitement, exultation, embarrassment, and then pity.

The dressing station witnessed an amazing tank battle at night at very close range, amidst a great MLRS barrage, as Iraqi tanks were ambushed while withdrawing northwards up a wadi.

Our entry into Kuwait on G+3 followed a gallop up a tapline road with enemy 'refugees' begging for food all along the way. We entered Kuwait only to be met with the sight of two CVR(T)s under fire to our front. A mad scramble forward soon elicited the information that it had been one of those unfortunate 'blue on blue' incidents and that, thankfully, no one had been killed.

By the time the ceasefire was announced we were grouped with several other regiments, poised near the Kuwait–Basra highway. It was amusing to hear the BBC World Service announce that there was silence on all fronts and at the same time to hear sporadic bursts of heavy gunfire.

The war ended with us eighteen kilometres NW of Kuwait City. Several teams were sent to assist the bomb disposal efforts in the city. A few enemy casualties with old wounds dribbled into the dressing station long after the cessation of hostilities.

All in all, we did not see too many harrowing sights, although most of us will retain some enduring, poignant memories. Most of us witnessed many good and positive things – teamwork, friendship, selflessness, and kindness.

From my own point of view, several criticisms could be laid at my door. The first that I heard was that I should have delegated much of the sharp-end work to a subordinate. My own feeling is that leaders are meant to set an example and inspire confidence. Whether or not I achieved that I'll never know.

My greatest regret is that, in trying to ensure that no favouritism was shown to anyone in the difficult desert conditions, I perhaps demanded too much self-reliance from my officers.

It was a great honour to command so many fine professional soldiers and to have been given such a challenging role. Every man played a vital part in the success of our mission, and I am acutely aware that my award of the MBE could perhaps best be summed up as 'Many Blokes' Efforts'.

A DENTIST'S EXPERIENCE IN THE GULF

[W. J. N. Collins, BDS, MSc, FDS, RCPS, called back into service during the Gulf War to help the hard-pressed regulars]

I was called upon to serve as second-in-command of an army hospital in Saudi Arabia during the recent Gulf War.

On leaving university in 1963, I joined the Royal Army Dental Corps, in which I served until 1979, retiring with the rank of Lt Colonel. On leaving the regular army, I joined the 205 Scottish General Hospital (V) and was still serving in that unit at the outbreak of the Gulf War. In late December 1990 this TA hospital was selected for service in the Gulf to reinforce the overstretched regular army medical services.

At the beginning of 1990 I had been asked by numerous friends and colleagues if there was any likelihood of my being conscripted back into the regular army. I was honestly of the opinion that there was no likelihood whatsoever! On December 20th I received a phone call inviting me to report for mobilisation on December 27th. Although mobilised on that date, we did not in fact leave Scotland until January 2nd. Even the Gulf War could not be allowed to interfere with the Scottish unit's New Year celebrations.

On receiving the telephone call, my initial reaction was one of disbelief. This was gradually replaced by apprehension about the uncertainties which lay ahead. My biggest disappointment, however, was that my oldest daughter, Lesley and her husband, Neil Woon Sam, both of whom are dentists in Trinidad, arrived home on December 21st to spend three weeks holiday with us. The all too infrequent times we spent together are very precious and I missed the last ten days of their holiday. Strangely, however, their presence at home made the farewell to Vanda, my wife, and my other daughter and son a little easier.

As members of the TA we had regularly undergone training in establishing a military hospital and in other aspects such as chemical warfare protection. However, we were given a week of intensive training, and it was not surprising that the impending war helped to concentrate the mind wonderfully. During this spell we also received more than a dozen different vaccinations against a bewildering variety of biological warfare agents.

On arrival at Riyadh, the capital city of Saudi Arabia, we set about creating a full general hospital, complete with 600 beds, operating theatres with ten tables and dental radiography, central sterilisation and pathology departments. This was all created in the shell of a newly-constructed airport terminal, without even the most basic supplies of power, water and drainage. The entire complex was brought to operational standard within ten days and was an enormous credit to the whole unit.

In the meantime, the air battle had begun and the unit was regularly and repeatedly in the Scud missile firing line. Since the hospital was situated next to the launching pads for the Patriot anti-missile missiles, we enjoyed some multi-million pound fireworks. We had two major things to be thankful for: very few Scud missiles managed to break through the Patriot defences, and, of course, none of them contained chemical agents. As a unit we suffered nothing more than the discomfort of long times spent in protective suits and respirators.

As everyone now appreciated, there were thankfully small numbers of allied casualties. While being delighted that we had so little clinical work to perform, there was inevitably a strange feeling of anti-climax, particularly among those surgeons and physicians who had volunteered to cope with large numbers of severely injured patients.

At the end of the land battle, we also realised that there were surprisingly few injured Iraqi soldiers and the unit was "stood down" within a few days.

We had a total of fourteen dentists serving in the unit. Apart from myself as second-in-command, there was one regular army maxillo-facial surgeon (Colonel David Boulton), three general duty dentists (Col Brian Toms and Capt. Mark Earl and Paul Grainger), and nine dentists employed as anaesthetic support officers (Lt Col Steve Monk, Majors Jane Berresford, Kate Fisher, Bob McCormick, Willie MacEachen, Maggie Softly, Hugh Tyrell and Captains Bernard Palmer and Cathie Sinclair).

One of the most exciting times was undoubtedly the first Scud missile, which was exploded directly above our heads. Certainly that night 'the earth moved' for us all! Another personal exciting memory is of the flight I had on one of the refuelling tankers which went up to the Iraqi borders to refuel the fighter bomber jets. To watch these heavily-laden planes refuelling almost within touching distance of the VC10 tanker in which we were flying was something I will long remember.

Of course, it was by no means all work in Riyadh. We had, for example, a Burns supper and a St David's Day party... both sadly lacking in alcohol! At the Burns supper I was just about to propose a toast to the immortal memory of Robert Burns when we had a Scud attack. Everyone climbed into full protective gear and flattened themselves on the floor. When it was all over, we carried on with celebration and the toast!

On March 9th (months before we dared hoped it was possible) the unit began its return to the United Kingdom. The first 300 were flown to Prestwick in Scotland and were greeted by pipe bands, government ministers, television and radio... and of course their families. As second-in-command, it was my unfortunate duty to remain behind and travel back with the very last group. We crept into Brize Norton in England, with the minimum of fuss or attention.

Looking back on it, the spell in the Gulf was an experience of a lifetime, although not one I would wish to repeat. We were fortunate to suffer no more than some inconvenience and personal discomforts, but how different it might have been!

OPERATION GRANBY: The Celler Rats logo

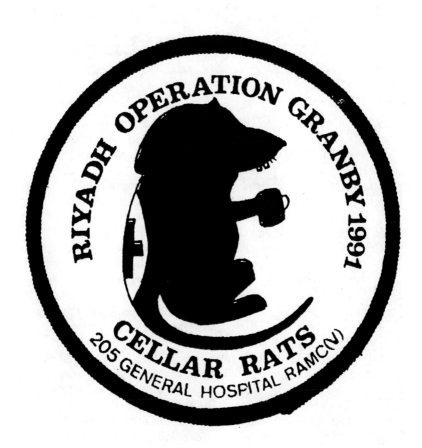

OPERATION GRANBY: A SANITARY TALE

[By Capt. C.A.E Jeffrey, RADC]

When I was asked to write a short article on my six months attachment with Dressing Station One Bravo, First Armoured Field Ambulance during Operation Granby, my mind began to produce wonderfully soft focus pictures of glorious advances at the head of a convoy of one ton ambulances, days of balmy sunshine filled with banter and intellectual stimuli, staggering vistas of the rugged yet serenely beautiful desert landscape... Then I thought – well, hold on a minute, has it really been that long since I was there?

Gradually with a conscious effort and a day spent dressed in a NBC training suit to capture the atmosphere again, the insidious soft focus began to harden and I could think honestly about my experiences. I have no doubt it was of great value to me and I am pleased to have been so involved in the largest movement of this great army of ours since World War Two. But, by heck, retrospect is a wonderful process which I'll try to avoid too much if I can.

I flew from Hamburg to Al Jubayl on 18th October 1990 and after a short stay in the infamous dockside sweat-sheds (while we awaited the arrival by sea of our vehicles and equipment) we moved out to our first desert location in the Al Fadili training area. I won't bore you with map references, routes, positions, logisitics, exercise details, casualty facts and figures – someone else will probably do that. Nor do I propose to talk about the actual ground advance through Southern Iraq and into Kuwait, which was abrupt, uncomfortable, fiercely interesting and exciting, not a bit frightening at times, and I think you've probably heard all about it. I'll just bore you with a little of what everyday life was like... yes, the focus is really getting sharper now!

We lived in a tent – myself, three of our medical officers (including one lady) and one of the nursing officers. It wasn't a bad tent but it was a tent nonetheless, and quite an old one at that, with many varied holes in it. These let the light out at night (in quantity and patterns that wouldn't have disgraced Blackpool in November!) which would have worried us had Iraq had an air force. As we discovered later, they also let in the rain, in vast quantities, highly disproportionate to the size of the holes – none of us could explain the physical principles behind this phenomenon.

In fact, it was quite amazing the rapidity with which the novelty of the rain in the desert wore off. I reckon rain in the desert to be marginally more unpleasant than rain in Europe, particularly in a mature canvas life-support unit (otherwise known as an ancient rotting, hole 12' × 12').

Other phenomenon encountered during life in Saudi Arabia included the incredible timing possessed by dental casualties. They did have an uncanny ability to arrive just as I was dipping my smalls into two inches of cold swimming pool water (everything was heavily chlorinated) in an attempt (vain, I must confess) to remove the charcoal grey tinge (à la NBC suit) from my once pristine white boxer shorts. Not once in five months did I successfully complete my full wash cycle!

My Dental Clerk Assistant, Cpl Adam Gzreskowiak, a very amiable, intelligent and able NCO, would poke his head through the tent flap or through the ubiquitous desert scrim (guaranteed to viciously snag one's combat suit bottoms, one's boots laces, one's hat, one's watch, even while appearing to be metres away from one) and, before I'd even given up trying to induce a semblance of a lather with my Travel Wash, would announce the arrival of half a dozen assorted gunners complete with assorted aches and pains.

Three hours later, after much screeching of overworked Technobox, much smoke from a overworked Technobox and much chemfil dispensed from rapidly dwindling private supply, I would stagger back into our tent to find the 'one and only basin' hijacked (never trust a medical officer) and my wet, but as yet unclean, smalls in a neat pile by my campcot. By the time the basin became vacant again, the same half a dozen squaddies were back again following their immediate consumption of three pounds of compo boiled sweets on the transport back to their unit.

220

It was the actual business of living as sanitarily as possible that was the most time-consuming part of the day (and night). There were the halcyon early days of virtually unlimited (but freezing cold even in the hottest period another desert phenomenon!) water supply and standing in the wooden showers where the November shrieks and wails gave way to December's and January's utter breathless silences (there is a level of cold which the body ceases to attempt to complain about, simply concentrating on allowing one's wedding tackle to remain as an appendage and not an internal organ).

These in turn gave way to more spartan days of a bucket shower running through a pierced compo skimmed milk tin. This operation involved the depressing experience of carrying a jerry can to the QM's department – where a constant party seemed to be going on involving tropical warmth from kerosene burners.

Unavailable to the rest of the army, coffee was served laced with more than compo dried skimmed milk and there were fresh rations, the like of which the EC food mountains would be embarrassed about. One then had to cajole and grovel with great eloquence (there is no point in bribing men who have everything!) to be allowed to fill said jerry can with extra-freezing cold swimming pool water. This was carried back where, with the help of a colleague, one let the string which held the bucket down, filled it and hoisted it up again, spilling most of the precious water as it went. One stripped sharpishly and, standing inside the 'one and only basin', flipped the 'on' lever to start the freezing dribble going.

As soon as one was damp, one switched off, soaped down (usually removing at least two layers of goose pimpled skin due to the sand stuck in the soap bar) and then (if one had been frugal enough) experienced the final luxurious rinse (luxurious relatively as by this stage one's whole body was completely numb!). One then used what was collected in the 'one and only basin' (not a pretty sight) to attempt to wash one's smalls in an operation which was inevitably interrupted by the head of Cpl Gzreskowiak appearing through the tent flap. Ah well! Déjà vu! It wasn't all unsuccessful wash days, however, not so.

As an honorary duty doctor's understudy, in an attempt to increase my medical knowledge and effectiveness as a resuscitation officer I spent many a happy hour dispensing drugs previously a world away from the DPF. This was not because my overworked Technobox had shuffled off this mortal coil or because the chemfil had run out; it was an extra duty and I did learn a great deal regarding basic examination procedures and minor surgery.

My illustrious GMP career was voluntarily curtailed when a military policeman, suffering from a severe and very red scrotal inflammation (the origins and treatment of which I was without a clue about and the examination of which I was going about somewhat warily), admitted a little caustically that I had dressed his cracked tooth four days previously and could he please see an MO about his bollocks!

I did, however, learn much from my RAMC colleagues (in particular Captains Mike Eaton and Roger Bramley) for which I was (and still am) very grateful. Their help, support, and friendship went a long way towards relieving my frantic worries as to how I would cope with mass battle trauma if and when it occurred. I can't go into detail here about every aspect of life during Operation Granby, but little thoughts do crop up all the times:

· ...of hours spent travelling in convoy in the wildly swinging enclosed box that is a one ton ambie and having nothing to look at except the lurid pornographic pictures with which the dubious RCT drivers had plastered the cabin, and nothing to think about except whether this crazy turn or the next would be our last – a bizarre experience that may well leave permanent mental scars!

· ...of having 2,500 toothbrushes stacked in boxes all round my bed which Messrs Stafford Miller posted to the DS in two sacks as tall as me in a response to a begging letter that I'd totally forgotten about.

· ...of vivid dreams about piping hot baths filled right up to the rim, pints of bitter, crisp salads, and other pleasurable things it's probably best to keep to myself.

· ...of smoke pouring out of a screeching Technobox!

· of my bed shaking for over thirty seconds, while more than thirty kilometres away a 15,000lb 'daisy cutter' bomb was being dropped on Iraqi defences.

· ....of frantic mood swings when letters from home (anywhere?) arrived or didn't.

· ...of the communal latrines where one tried at all costs to avoid going at the same time as Sgt Pepe, who invariably sat right next to you (admittedly he had little choice in the matter) and who was hilariously interested in bowel noises of any nature, either his own or anyone else's.

· ...of vain but valiant attempts in the early hot period to consume the specified fifteen litres of bottled water per day resulting in forays to the desert rising hourly (my kidneys never had it so good!).

The British Army alone must have raised Saudi Arabia's water table a couple of feet.

I returned to Germany by Kuwaiti Airline's Jumbo on 13th March 1991 and was fortunate enough to be met by Lt Col John Davies RADC and his wife Midge, who had had the brilliance and selflessness to bring out my girlfriend (now fiancée) Katy from London to meet me at Hanover Airport. I knew nothing of this.

I hadn't seen Katy for nearly six months, and although we had written avidly to each other we had only spoken three times by phone over that whole time. Needless to say, I almost forgot my luggage! Those two wonderful people gave us the run of the quarter that night – I still don't know where they disappeared to – and for such kindness I will always be grateful. Half a glass of champagne later I had to sit down before I fell down. I had endless fun tapping all four walls of the room without feeling them flapping.

Unfortunately, the death of a dream did occur as Col John had forgotten to put his water heater on and the longed-for 'hot bath right up to the neck' turned out to be disappointingly tepid. However, another half a glass of champagne and it didn't seem so important. I was home.

On a serious note to finish, thankfully as a DS with the Artillery Brigade we saw many fewer casualties than we had anticipated. Those we did see were dealt with compassionately, competently and were passed on quickly down the chain of evacuation. We all worked much harder clinically in the phases prior and subsequent to the ground assault, performing routine MRS functions including treatment of dental sick.

At these times the forward DS was, I feel, a most valuable medical support asset. The role as a dental/resuscitation officer in the DS is, I think, a very important one and one which we are trained rudimentarily for at best. I had never seen (let alone operated) a field dental set prior to October 1990. Most formal resuscitation training was snippets picked up from anaesthetists in the cosy, comfortable chats in calm sterile surroundings of ASRO courses.

Perhaps those primed for this role should have a little more formalised training – the BATLS course is a must, particularly as the Granby experience has rewritten much of CTRs. The most important thing for us as dental officers is not to undervalue ourselves. We know the basics, we can learn quickly, our manual dexterity is a practical asset not to be sniffed at.

The Field Ambulance dental officer role is one we should encourage, particularly as ASRO training (or CASO as it is now) becomes more selective. It is a role in which we can be very effective and ensure the continuing importance of the RADC in the Army Medical Support. I can feel the focus going blurry around the edges again... Glorious days!

CROATIA – OPERATION GRAPPLE

[Major C. A. E. Jeffrey, RADC]

As the Royal Fleet Auxiliary (RFA) ship *Sir Bedivere*, landing-ship logistic, edged ponderously into its berth at the harbour in Split, Croatia on 17th October 1992, I looked down at the small reception committee looking up at us and then turned my attention outwards to the abruptly rising mountains of the Adriatic coast. I wondered what exactly lay beyond. It was all as clear as mud at this stage.

A phone call was made to Dental Centre Woolwich and three days notice given to move to Twenty-Two Field Hospital RAMC Aldershot. A crack of dawn departure for Germany on what has to be the longest coach journey I have ever experienced (in an army bus too – no nice comfy seats, as you can imagine).

What followed was five days of chaos flitting from one transit accommodation dormitory to another – interspersed with lectures on mines awareness, weapons training, etc. Then finally the twelve day Mediterranean cruise from Emden to Split via Southampton and Gibraltar (a pity none of this qualified for airmiles!)

We were finally here – 'we' being the personnel of Medical Support Troop (MST). The Dental Detachment comprised myself and Pte P. S. Wood, RADC – a recent recruit to the Dental Corps but with five years infantry experience behind him. I had already nominated him for any trench digging or sandbagging that might become necessary.

We had been informed that we were to set up a mobile dental facility based at one of the four British locations. It was initially suggested to me that this should be Tomislavgrad (TSG) with the HQ of the National Support Element (NSE), but I personally felt that Vitez

LINE MAP – Danger Area

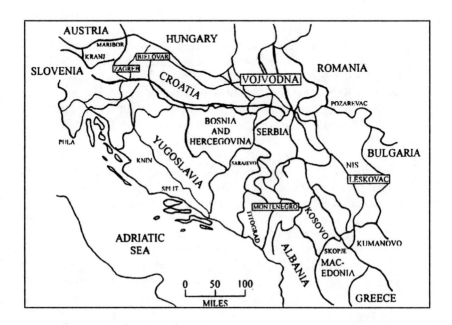

was to be preferred due to: *(a)* the presence there of MST-B who had all the supporting facilities I could possible wish for – including: transport, administration, resupply, x-ray, dispensary, theatre, wards and so on; and *(b)* the greatest single troop concentration with the presence of one Cheshire plus support.

There were as yet very few people in theatre when we arrived in Split and recces were still proceeding. We knew we were to move up country but probably not for at least a week to ten days. Therefore we all had a trial run at setting up on board the *Sir Bedivere*, with ourselves in the ship's hospital.

We had figured out how the field kit actually went together and sorted out one or two teething troubles (oops!). With the generous help of the ship's engineer, we began to treat our first patients Navy-style (but better, of course!).

On 4th November the MST packed up and made the long and winding trip to Vitez. This was our first foray into the interior, and the change was noticeable. The Adriatic coastal belt is very narrow, with a range of mountains descending directly into the sea in some places. At first we seemed to go up and up without check.

The former Yugoslavian inland (and especially Bosnia-Herzegovina) is indeed a very mountainous region – bleak, majestic and beautiful, with a low density population living in small settlements of often very basically built houses. Pine forests abound, fast-flowing rivers go by, lush green meadows stretch away to please the eye.

One can definitely imagine groups of partisans in World War Two hiding out from the frustrated forces of the Third Reich. The people are brown, weatherbeaten, tough-looking individuals with prematurely lined faces but with strong backs that still carry impossible loads of wood from the forests to home. The Muslims can be detected usually by their darker colouring and the gaily-coloured dresses of the women – complete with yashmak in many cases.

Children are everywhere, and they became a constant feature of the following months, lining the roads (even in the most bitter of temperatures) in the hope of some sweets or chocolate tossed from the cab of a four-tonner or a UN Land Rover. Indeed the British Army and other UN soldiers must be responsible for a fair old bit of dental deterioration in kids who already had a severe caries problem. I didn't have time to stop and give succour.

The traveller in Bosnia/Croatia passes through innumerable checkpoints manned by militiamen of many and varied factions depending on the dominating local warlord. Seldom were we molested over the tour beyond drunken abuse or the occasional shot into the car (still enough the first time to make me glad of my seat-belt!). By and large, UK vehicles were allowed free passage unless there was a fight going on in the vicinity.

Anyway... on reaching Vitez we were introduced to the school which was to become home to the MST for nearly four months. Two classrooms were set aside to house the ward and operating theatre. We set up our wares in a corner of the ward and very quickly began to find ourselves busy.

The dental detachment obviously had a responsibility for all the British troops in Bosnia/Croatia and so the question of transport had to be tackled. The MST had only one Land Rover, one ambulance and one four ton truck, all of which were constantly in use. Initially I was *generously* donated a trailer (please note, heavy sarcasm) in which Woody and I were supposed to pack all our personal and dental kit and hitch rides from posh people between locations! With some scepticism I tried this and very quickly over the next week vowed I would never do it again!

Fortunately a Land Rover became available from HQ NSE and we immediately pasted an RADC sticker on to the side and adopted it. To do the driving I was lucky to be able to poach one of the MST medical technicians (CMT), Lcpl Shirley RAMC, who also in the event became a very effective Dental Support Specialist (DSS) back-up to Pte Wood. That was it – the Balkans' Independent Dental Expeditionary Troop (the BIDET!) had been formed. We were mobile (albeit not upwardly!).

From that point life became easier. We would spend approximately one week in Vitez treating, as well as our own troops, those of the Dutch Transport Battalion, French Engineer Regiment, and the various nationalities of the UN HQ in Kiseliak. Even the odd aid-worker or pressman slipped in if they were having problems. We would then pack up (the kit fitting into one large and two medium Lacon boxes) and drive off into the sunset for about a week's round trip of Gornji Vakuf (GV), TEG and Split.

Each trip was eventful – not just because of prevailing weather and road conditions, which often cut Vitez off entirely from the outside world. Fighting in GV or Mostar often dictated our route and, more than once, hard miles had to be retraced to find alternative ways through. Blown up bridges, Serbian bombardments, snow and ice all played their part. At least we didn't have to worry about the M25!

One evening in the British base at TSG we were 'privileged' to receive about 150 incoming artillery shells in close vicinity, the next door building belonging to the Engineers taking two direct hits. A night in the bomb shelter with 100 troops was not the ideal prelude to the next day's dental list.

On one trip to a blocked road, as part of a two-vehicle only convoy, we suddenly became the object of interest for seventy or eighty Croatian 'Blackshirts' of the fascist 'HOS', who appeared *en masse* to investigate the hold up. The unnerving looking men, armed absolutely to the teeth, proceeded to bombard us with snowballs as we tried to negotiate delicately past the wreckage of a Dutch truck. We felt that retaliation would be churlish and the three of us just smiled and waved through the onslaught.

We were certainly busy – 650 patients were treated (332 of those presenting with some form of pain) – and the field kit proved very adequate. A few deficiencies existed, notably x-ray and sterilisation equipment, but the units that we possessed had gained our respect as being hardwearing, portable and adaptable.

On 20th February the MST moved out of the school and into a purpose-built prefabricated 'hospital' complex. Dental Centre Vitez was born also – an individual portacabin situated next to the MST. Our own space, electricity with a bit more reliability than the local grid, windows (albeit with no view), and even wall-to-wall carpeting!

Operation Grapple certainly showed a definite need for dental cover on out-of-area operations, as well as proving the ability of the RADC to now provide a genuinely peripatetic service over the most difficult terrain. This surely is something no one could argue a case for civilisation of... (Cue the grey man in Whitehall with some fatuous remark about the Territorial Army!)

At all locations and by all the UN nations present we were well received and most were (I hope) happily surprised at the refined standard of the service available. I could not have asked for better travelling companions and assistance than I got in Pte Wood and LCpl Shirley. These two epitomised the sense of humour and capacity for graft of the British soldier. In the same vein, the MST as a whole were a friendly and helpful bunch who welcomed their dental 'satellite' into the fold very readily.

Our six months came to an end with the arrival of Capt. Paul Grainger and LCpl Conibeere, RADC, on 31st March. I wish them luck and a safe journey. It was definitely getting warmer. At least (in more ways than one perhaps!) Operation Grapple may well be on the postings plot for some time to come.

CROATIA – OPERATION HANWOOD
[Major J. M. R. Preece, RADC]

Imagine sitting in a basement that is slowly filling up with smoke, listening to the clump of exploding rounds, the crack of small fire arms and the horrendous scream of jet engines just overhead. Suddenly there is an enormous explosion and somebody shouts, "Everybody out." As shadowy figures stumble through the fog towards the dubious safety of daylight your job is to check that the basement rooms are empty. "Room clear!" you shout as you career up the steps emerging into bright sunlight.

The sight that greets your eyes is a landscape from hell – billowing smoke, a burning tank, broken bodies, some whimpering, others are still. Green figures are running around shouting, "Medic!" or, "Over here!" In a pile of rubble you hear the ominous clanking of heavy armour. Suddenly you come upon a camera crew filming two medics trying to resuscitate a bloodied body. Where is Kate Adie? Where are you? The Somme? Normandy? Goose Green? Los Angeles?

No... It is Copehill Down FIBUA village on Salisbury Plain! As the smoke clears and the noise level descends to something like normal you see the bodies 'rise up' and light a cigarette. You see the traumatised amputee grow an arm and curse saying, "Did you see how low those idiots were flying?"

Why is the dental officer sitting (or running and coughing his lungs up) through all this? Well, pull up a sandbag and I'll tell you.

In February 1992, having just returned from Exercise Lion Sun in Cyprus, Twenty-Four (Airmobile) Field Ambulance RAMC was warned off for deployment to Croatia, as part of the British contribution to the United Nations Peace Keeping force (UNPROFOR) in the former Yugoslavia.

The unit, along with elements of Thirty Signal Regiment, a REME Workshops, RE, ACC RMP EFI, RAChD, RCT, were to make up the British Medical Battalion, or BRITMEDBAT in 'UN speak'.

Preparations began immediately: ordering stores, flak jackets, bullet-proof white paint, and all the necessary paraphernalia of war in peace. Preparing for all the eventualities, we were run through all imaginable scenarios from security to mine clearing to all-out war. (If anyone reading this is the least bit nervous of load noises, I recommend you don't do the Copehill Down package!) The only thing we didn't experience was death by cirrhosis! (Honestly!)

Come March, the advance party had just got on the 'bus' when everything ground to a halt, so that John Major could have an election. Two months later it was back on the 'bus'.

During Operation Granby (the Gulf War) I formed some interesting opinions about the state of the field dental kit scalings, and so, when I was going on Operation Hanwood for six months, I did the only reasonable thing – and tore them up. Because of the political pause I was able, by fair means and foul, to build what I considered a reasonable dental set-up.

After some verbal 'crowbarring' I managed to secure the Field Surgical Team (FST) dental kit from Defence Medical Equipment Depot, (DMED) Ludgershall, only to discover some remarkable deficiencies such as no amalgamator (Why? Because no amalgam is supplied?) the facility for internal fibre-optic couplings but only standard hand pieces, no x-ray facilities, etc.

Before the CO DMED starts writing my Court Martial I must thank him and his staff quite unreservedly for all the hard work and co-operation they gave me in converting my nightmare into a 'dream' dental set-up.

Our eventual arrival in the theatre had shades of Granby. Flying to an airport, driving for hours in a dilapidated coach, and finally being dumped in an aircraft hanger – does this ring any bells? This was our first experience of Pleso Airbase, Zagreb – HQ for the next six months.

The first priority was the preparation and dispersal of the sector medical teams to their allotted 'outposts', and then the very dirty job of cleaning up the mess left behind by the departing JNA (Yugoslav National Army). We were still doing this six months later.

As BRITMEDBAT began getting organised, it was time for dentistry to rear its head again. A call from Knin in sector south sent me gallivanting off with my emergency kit to sunnier Serbian climes, leaving my faithful sidekick, Cpl Adrian (Dimmy) Dimitrio, to carry on sorting out the detritus of modern dentistry. Another life saved and I returned triumphant (*back in time for tea and medals*, I think the expression is), only to find that I had been 'organised' during my absence.

A book had appeared along with fat faces, absent amalgams, and halitosis hygiene. I noticed in relief and professional pride in my colleagues that the majority were not wearing British uniforms.

So began six months of international dentistry. Both Cpl Dimitrio and I became masters in sign language and the very British form of address when speaking to a foreigner – speaking loudly and slowly.

During this time relations with our erstwhile adversaries from the Warsaw Pact were firmly cemented. Czechs threw us in rivers, Russians prescribed vodka for our ills, and Ukrainians declared undying devotion to the Union Flag.

By accident Cpl Dimitrio and I managed to reinvent the wheel. Having decided that Zagreb was growing stale (the atmosphere, not the beer) the Dental Duo planned escape. We packed all of our kit into a Land Rover and drove off into the sunset, setting up in various locations over the four United Nations Protected Areas (UNPAS) where the British were stationed.

The ability to move a complete dental set-up, including x-ray machine, portable darkroom, high speed fibre optic drills, light cure machine, compressor, Little Sister steriliser, and all the necessary consumables, was a great success, although we did raise a few eyebrows in the warm weather when our uniform comprised only a tunic and a pair of shorts! Thus the mobile dental team was restored.

During the closing months of our tour Operation Grapple became headline news and we Hanwoodians began to think of ourselves as the forgotten army. The Sappers, having been perforated in Sarajevo and brassed off by the French, decided to go and drink their Guinness elsewhere, much to the relief of the civilian helicopter pilots (but that's another story). The Signals were filtering away to Split and all the bigwigs only stopped at Zagreb to catch a plane home. Even 'P Info' decided it was more fun to dodge rounds on the road to Vitez.

We did have one visitor who was very welcome – Capt. (now Major) Craig Jeffrey, RADC, popped into say hello. He picked the night of our Guy Fawkes celebrations, obviously in preparation for his Grapple experiences.

Finally November turned to December and our thoughts turned to home. Four (Armoured) Field Ambulance were on their way to replace us, bringing Capt. Neil McKenzie to replace me, to sort out all the problems only half solved during our time. (Sorry, Neil, I didn't know about Belgrade.)

If only one thing comes out of my time in Croatia, I hope it will be the demonstration that mobile dentistry is something we need to equip for, because it is very rewarding and very much appreciated by those on the receiving end (for a change!).

Finally I would like to extend my thanks to all who helped me during my tour, especially Cpl Dimitrio, who kept me on the straight and narrow, and Flt Lt Karen Horsham and her team at DMED, and the 'Home Front' back at Dental Centre Catterick.

Printed in the United Kingdom
by Lightning Source UK Ltd.
99750UKS00001B/154-159